NEANDERTHIN

Eat Like a Caveman to Achieve a Lean, Strong, Healthy Body

RAY AUDETTE
WITH TROY GILCHRIST

FOREWORD BY
MICHAEL R. EADES, M.D.

ST. MARTIN'S PRESS ❧ NEW YORK

Book Design by Kathryn Parise

Library of Congress Cataloging-in-Publication Data

Audette, Ray V.
    Neanderthin : eat like a caveman to achieve a lean, strong,
healthy body / Ray Audette, Troy Gilchrist.
      p. cm.
    Includes bibliographical references (p.).
    ISBN 0-312-24338-3
    1. Low-carbohydrate diet. 2. Prehistoric peoples—Food.
I. Gilchrist, Troy. II. Title.
RM237.73.A86 1999
613.2'6—dc21   99-36356
                                                CIP

10 9 8 7 6 5 4 3 2

FOR

Grayson Haak Audette
Who, while just a spirit,
caused this book to be written

AND

Renee E. Solinger
Loving wife and spiritual inspiration

Author's Note

This book is for informational purposes only. Readers should consult a doctor before making any major change in diet.

CONTENTS

ACKNOWLEDGMENTS

As I am not a doctor or a scientist, I have benefited greatly from many in-depth conversations with each of the following people: Dr. Alan S. Brown, Dr. Michael R. Eades, Dr. Vaughn Bryant of Texas A&M University, Dr. S. Boyd Eaton of Emory University, and Dr. Loren Cordain of Colorado State University. Without the contributions each made to the research process of which this book is the final product, *NeanderThin* would not have been possible. I am grateful to each for his contribution. Thanks also to editor Heather Jackson of St. Martin's Press, literary agent Jim Donovan, and Jeff Scroggins for his culinary expertise and recipes.

FOREWORD

With the invention of agriculture, the composition of man's diet changed. Where Paleolithic (Old Stone Age) humans had derived most of their energy from foods rich in protein and fat and low in carbohydrates, Neolithic people began to rely on diets high in carbohydrates and low in fat and protein. The disastrous ramifications of this reversal for human health and longevity are recorded in the remains of bodies from the Neolithic period.

You may be thinking, This is all very interesting, but who cares? Maybe it doesn't make a rat's behind's worth of difference whether we eat meat, vegetables, or Purina Monkey Chow as long as we get enough vitamins, minerals, and other nutrients. So what if we have the same basic body structure, both outwardly and inwardly, that we had 50,000 years ago? We ate some plant foods then; we obviously had (and have) whatever it takes digestively to deal with them—so what's the problem with our eating less meat and more carbohydrate-rich plant foods?

In answering these questions, let me point out a couple of facts that you may not have considered: First, just because our physiology can handle a small dose of something doesn't mean that it can deal with a large dose of the same thing without problems developing. For example, we have all the enzymes necessary to deal with alcohol in moderate dosages, but anyone who has overindulged knows what happens when we get too much.

Second, when we talk about primitive man eating plant foods, we're not talking about the same plant foods you and I eat. Go out in the woods and pick some wild crabapples or wild cherries, dig up a few roots, gather some nuts and seeds, and find some tender shoots. Harvest this bounty, take it home, and lay it out on the table—these, and wild foods like them, are the ones that were available to our primitive ancestors. Now, go to the grocery store and bring home a sack of the fruits and vegetables you find there. Put them beside your harvest of wild foods. You will very quickly see that the plant foods available to us, after thousands of generations of hybridization to increase sugar and starch content and to decrease fiber content, are very different from the plant foods available to Paleolithic humans. The plant foods our ancestors ate prior to the development of agriculture were nutrient-dense, not particularly high in carbohydrates, and contained much more fiber than today's fruits and vegetables.

The main problem with our modern, civilized diet is that it provides us with abnormal quantities of the various nutrients we need to sustain our health. In nature, humans eat a diet low in carbohydrates, high in protein, and relatively high in fat. In contrast, our modern diet tends to be very high in carbohydrates, with percentages of dietary protein and fat varying by nation and culture. The result of this shift in our diet has been the rise of degenerative diseases that were unknown to our Paleolithic ancestors.

As a result of our research into Paleolithic nutrition, my wife, Mary Dan Eades, and I, both medical doctors, developed a low-carbohydrate, high-protein eating program that we have detailed in our book *Protein Power*. Our program is very similar to that advocated by Ray Audette in *NeanderThin*. Although the "NeanderThin" approach is more restrictive than we have found to be necessary for our patients, this book is well written and offers a unique perspective on the subject of Paleolithic nutrition. Ray Audette writes from the position of a layperson who researched and adopted the Paleolithic diet and lifestyle in response to his own serious health problems (diabetes and rheumatoid arthritis), which disappeared after he became "NeanderThin." In his research Ray relied heavily on peer-reviewed scientific literature written by doctors, anthropologists, and archaeologists. But you won't find phrases like "exploiting mobile resources" in this book. His writing is clear and understandable to the average person. He brings the science of Paleolithic health and nutrition down to earth.

As a medical doctor who has prescribed a very similar eating program for more than 5,000 patients, I feel comfortable in recommending *NeanderThin* to anyone interested in losing weight, lowering blood pressure and serum cholesterol, controlling diabetes, and improving overall health and fitness.

—Michael R. Eades, M.D.,
Coauthor of Protein Power

INTRODUCTION

I first met Ray Audette when we were both nine years old. He had just transferred into my fourth-grade class and came to my house for his first Cub Scout meeting. Ray was fascinated by my collection of bird nests, shells, insects, and butterflies. When he found out that my father kept a menagerie in the waiting room of his orthodontia clinic, Ray was hooked. After learning that my after-school chores consisted of caring for this little zoo, Ray appointed himself my assistant and best friend.

Every day after school when other boys played sandlot sports, Ray and I would feed the animals, clean the fish tanks, and collect new specimens from the local ponds and woods to fill the terrariums and aquariums. In between these endeavors we would study nature and conduct experiments. Thus it was that I conducted my first X-ray experiments (the effects of dental X-rays on marigold seeds) and surgery (compound fracture of a pigeon wing) with Ray by my side.

In many ways we were very similar. We both kept falcons. We were both well read for our age (they didn't call us nerds then, though they might today). In the summer of the fifth grade I went to a school for gifted children, and Ray went to high school. I took up the clarinet, and Ray took up the violin. I wasn't a good athlete, and when we chose sides for sports, Ray was always chosen after me. We were very close for several years. Eventually, Ray moved to Texas to study philosophy, and I remained in New York to begin my medical education. We drifted apart and didn't keep in touch.

I was, therefore, very surprised when, twenty-five years later, I received an overnight package containing the manuscript of this book. I was even more surprised when Ray informed me by phone that the NeanderThin program was partially inspired by my own experience with food allergies. Since childhood I have been severely allergic to wheat, corn, soybeans, chocolate, eggs, nuts, and fish. According to Ray, my own ability to cope with these dietary restrictions under any circumstances gave him the confidence to give up the staple foods of modern life.

Naturally I read his book immediately. I found it well written and not filled with the usual medical jargon. It's entertaining and in places displays great wit. More important, this work represents a paradigm shift in our views of nutrition and obesity. Ray's beliefs in a natural diet are purely logical. His view of obesity as an immune system response to foods introduced by technology is revolutionary.

Whether the reader is a physician or layperson my professional advice is the same: Take two tablets (see the Ten Commandments at the end of Chapter 7), and call on your local library to check out Ray's references as I have done. As most of these references are peer-reviewed sources, they contain well-researched and accurate information. Through their own references the articles and books listed in the Bibliography also make good starting points for further research.

After seeing your own results and reading the literature, I'm sure you will agree, as I do, with the principles of *NeanderThin*. Happy hunting and gathering!

—*Alan S. Brown, M.D.*

DR. ALAN S. BROWN is a physician in Springfield, Massachusetts, where he practices radiology and Paleolithic nutrition. He received his undergraduate degree from Clark University in Wooster, Massachusetts, and his Doctor of Medicine degree from Brown University. Dr. Brown is also an active member of the American Medical Association and the American Board of Radiology.

FIRST LAW

Do not eat the fruit of the technology*
that makes edible [†] the inedible.^{††}

—GENESIS 2:17

---

*English for "tree of knowledge" from the Greek *tech* (weave) and *nology* (of knowledge).

[†] In ancient Hebrew, synonymous with "good."

^{††} In ancient Hebrew, synonymous with "evil."

PART ONE

Understanding the
Precepts of a
Paleolithic Diet

CHAPTER ONE

A History of Dieting

As with any living creatures, humans must be constantly concerned with food. No matter what else occupies our time and efforts, we must eat to survive. Our preoccupation with eating is expressed in the prehistoric record in the forms of tools used in obtaining food and cave art depictions of hunting strategies. Even the most primitive of preliterate human tribes has food taboos in its oral traditions. Some of the most ancient of writings are the traditional scriptures of the great world religions. In all of these we can find the prohibition or recommendation of many kinds of foods. Dietary rules vary from religion to religion according to the agricultural practices of the geographical regions involved. These philosophies have continued to evolve as problems produced by new technologies have made new forms of civilization necessary.

Ancient civilizations were models of economic efficiency. By using simple inventions such as the plow, metalwork, and sailing ships, they were able to dominate the known world. These civilizations fell in turn as they reached the technological limits of both their productivity and their armies.

Our current interest in diet is rooted in the Industrial Revolution and its effects on the diet and lifestyle of nineteenth-century humans.

In the early nineteenth century, people moved from farms to cities to work in the new factories made possible by the invention of steam power. As urban population densities grew, feeding the new workers became difficult. These displaced farmers no longer lived where their food was produced, so new methods of food preparation, preservation, transportation, and distribution were required.

Inventors and entrepreneurs were quick to rise to the occasion with solutions to the problems of mass food production. Steam-powered mills began to produce white flour, which had a much longer shelf life than previous whole grain products. Bottled food, perfected by Napoleon for his conquests, soon gave way to canned foods using the same techniques. Traditional methods of salting and curing meat were modified to allow mass production. And for the first time, chemical preservatives were added to extend the shelf life of foods. With the advent of new processing technologies, food could be mass-produced at a central location and transported by newly invented, steam-powered boats and trains to almost any place in the known world. Grocery stores and restaurants were established to sell these food products wherever people lived.

While the new commercially produced foods were inexpensive and plentiful, the traditional farm fare of fresh meat, fruits, and vegetables did not become affordable or accessible to the average city dweller until the twentieth-century invention of refrigeration. Urban populations came to depend on baked goods prepared locally, imported flour, processed meats (salted, cured, and canned), and canned or pickled fruits and vegetables. Fresh foods, such as fruit or poultry or fresh ham, were reserved for Sundays if you were comfortably middle class or Christmas if you were part of the working class.

The trend toward manufactured foods was to spread even to the countryside. Farmers found that by eating store-bought foods they could concentrate their resources and efforts on raising fewer crops with a resulting increase in productivity and profits.

Without a revolution in food, the Industrial Revolution and the resulting urbanization of even remote towns would not have been possible in such a short period of time. But this change came at the cost of human health. People began to experience severe digestive problems and increasing obesity in the 1800s. Dyspepsia became one of the most common ailments diagnosed by doctors. Doctors also began to diagnose certain diseases for the first time, including rheumatoid arthritis and multiple sclerosis (MS). Various vitamin deficiencies (pellagra, scurvy, etc.) also became endemic even in rural populations.

Faced with the nineteenth-century doctor's relative disinterest in nutrition, the inventive minds of this period came forward to fill the void of wisdom concerning health and nutrition. Many colorful characters emerged during the 1800s offering cures for the national case of dyspepsia.

One of the first to stress the inseparable connection between diet and health was Sylvester Graham (of Graham cracker fame). Graham advocated a vegetarian diet with an emphasis on whole grains and fresh, raw fruits and vegetables. Through his lectures he became a national figure. And given the unavailability of fresh meat and the deplorable state of meatpacking plants during this time, it's no wonder that his program helped many to improve their health.

Weight loss was another problem waiting to be addressed by a talented amateur. In the 1840s an English businessman named William Banting became concerned about his increasing obesity. After consulting Dr. William Harvey, Banting began to reduce the amount of starch and sugar in his diet, arriving at what today we would call a low-carbohydrate diet. His subsequent success in reducing his considerable girth led him to write the world's first book on diet and weight loss. Banting's *Letter on Corpulence* was a bestseller for several decades.

Acting on a revelation from God in 1863, Sister Ellen White, founder of the Seventh-Day Adventist Church, led her followers to consume a vegetarian diet that incorporated many of the same foods as Graham's diet. Sister White and her husband subsidized the medical education of one of their young followers and helped him establish a health resort in the Adventist hometown of Battle Creek, Michigan. Dr. John Harvey Kellogg opened his sanitarium in 1876. A proponent of what he called "biologic" living, Kellogg's prescribed treatments of electroshock, light baths, hydrotherapy (baths, saunas, etc.), and five-gallon yogurt enemas would be considered of questionable value today. Nevertheless, Kellogg's temple of health, called "the San," was considered the most advanced institution of its kind both nationally and internationally.

Ever-increasing numbers of patrons were exposed to a gleaming white facility that closely resembled the health spas of today. Its rooms were filled with newly invented exercise machines and groups performing calisthenics and laughing exercises. Steam baths, saunas, vapor rooms, and swimming facilities were available. Results were measured by the latest testing equipment, which was used to examine muscle development, lung power, body fat, and the chemical composition of all the body's waste products.

The menu at the San would evoke a sense of *déjà vu* in anyone familiar with the USDA's food pyramid. Kellogg advocated a low-fat, high-complex-carbohydrate, high-fiber diet. Meat, especially red meat, was to be avoided at all times, and Kellogg's research labs invented several protein substitutes, including many forms of breakfast cereal, peanut butter, and soy and yogurt concoctions. These were served to patrons in carefully measured portions. When the technology for measuring food nutrient composition became available, patrons were provided menus with fat, carbohydrate, protein, and fiber quantity listings similar to the labels on today's food packaging.

Although weight loss was not an overwhelming concern of Dr. Kellogg's (he was a very fat man), he recommended reducing calorie and fat consumption to his patients who wished to lose weight.

His program also required increasing indigestible fiber intake to encourage frequent defecation (three or four times daily). Combining the San's intensive dietary and exercise programs, many patients achieved significant weight loss. But the difficulty of maintaining the Kellogg regimen led to many repeat visits by inmates of the sanitarium.

Dr. Kellogg wrote over 200 articles and 81 books and performed over 22,000 operations before his death in 1943. This impressive body of work, along with the Kellogg Foundation established by his brother W. K. Kellogg, provided the basis for contemporary nutritional thinking.

Lulu Hunt, another harbinger of today's common dietary wisdom, used the precise methodology pioneered by Kellogg to introduce a new measure of food value to the overweight public. Published in 1918, her book *Diet and Health with Key to the Calories* recommended the 1,200-calorie, low-fat, high-carbohydrate diet familiar today to even the most casual follower of diets.

Others, however, were following in the footsteps of Banting. In 1888 James Salisbury published a diet book that recommended a low-carbohydrate regimen. To make cheap cuts of range-fed Texas beef more palatable, he recommended that they be ground and mixed with fat. The "Salisbury steak" lacked only the bun and garnishes of today's hamburger.

Vilhjalmur Stefansson:
Pioneer of Stone Age Nutrition

Born to Icelandic parents in a frontier town in Canada, Vilhjalmur Stefansson was famous in the earlier part of the twentieth century for his Arctic explorations. After a brief career as a cowboy, he became an anthropologist and studied at Harvard University. Through Harvard connections he received his first opportunity to go to the Arctic in 1906.

As his first expedition involved a long sea voyage and Stefansson was prone to seasickness, he offered to journey to the base camp in the Canadian Arctic by the overland route. Arriving in the fall at the mouth of the McKenzie River, he was dismayed to learn that the ship carrying the expedition team and supplies had been frozen at sea hundreds of miles away. With only the three-piece suit he had worn on the trip from Cambridge, he had to make plans for the winter. Stefansson's calling as an anthropologist led him to refuse the charity of the few white men in the area; instead, he moved in with an Eskimo family. He lived in their home, adopted their style of clothing, hunted with them, and ate their food.

These lessons would serve Stefansson well in his future career as an Arctic explorer and lecturer. While other explorers depended on tons of stored food and equipment, Stefansson needed only his rifle and the knowledge given him by the natives to probe the northernmost reaches of this unknown world. In expedition after expedition he gained greater and greater fame as the last white man to discover new land in the Americas and meet Eskimo who had no previous contact with civilization.

In between expeditions Stefansson went on lecture tours, and with his strange eating habits, he garnered much attention. Having adopted the Eskimo diet during his 1906 expedition, he saw no reason to give it up. This meant that he never ate vegetables. In the age of Kellogg this was thought to be impossible, so in 1929 Stefansson and a fellow explorer submitted to a one-year scientific study at a New York hospital to determine the effects of an all meat and high-fat diet on their bodies. Surprisingly, doctors and researchers found they thrived on it. (See Stefansson Studies section in Bibliography.)

Stefansson maintained his Eskimo diet until he was sixty and married a woman half his age. According to his autobiography, she tempted him with desserts and fancy baking until he began to eat in an almost civilized manner.

After eleven years of this domestic bliss, Stefansson suffered a minor stroke in 1960. During his convalescence he resumed what he called his Stone Age diet. After an almost complete recovery, he wrote his book *Cancer: Disease of Civilization,* in which he described the lack of what we now know to be autoimmune disorders among primitive, Stone Age peoples as discovered by himself and other explorers, missionaries, and seafarers throughout history.

During World War II, scientists working for governments on both sides had access to new kinds of lab animals: millions of military conscripts and concentration camp prisoners. By carefully controlling rations and monitoring the results they were able to formulate how to feed people as cheaply (and profitably) as possible. They were also able to determine what vitamins and other supplements were necessary to keep starving people working productively in slave labor factories and on the battlefield.

After the war this data was collected (often for only the price of a one-way ticket to Argentina) and used to formulate many new caloric-reduction diets, as well as vitamin and mineral supplements. New standards for manufactured foods required the addition of supplements to make up for deficiencies inherent to them. The U.S. Department of Agriculture was charged with regulating these new standards and issuing recommendations.

Stefansson experimented with all-meat diets during World War II, while advocating pemmican (a dehydrated and powdered raw meat and fat dish requiring no refrigeration) as a military ration. The U.S. Army never accepted his recommendation (ironically, German Luftwaffe pilots used it in their survival kits). His work did, however, inspire many new low-carbohydrate diets. Some of these in the 1950s recommended nothing but meat, fat, and water. None, however, were recommended or approved by either the government or the medical establishment. And though all of these diets used the results of Stefansson's work, none included his anthropological slant, which is crucial to understanding how low-carbohydrate diets affect the human body.

R. Buckminster Fuller is famous for inventing the geodesic dome, but most who know of his work are unaware that he advocated a diet of meat, vegetables, and fruit. In the 1960s, Bucky found himself very overweight—at five feet, five inches he weighed 200 pounds. Concerned about his increasing size, he applied his scientific and philosophic genius to the problem. His solution was, and remains, unique among low-carbohydrate diet advocates.

One of the basic tenets of Bucky Fuller's philosophy is that nature is always most efficient in using energy. The sun is Earth's main source of energy, and solar energy is directly concentrated in the form of plants through the process of photosynthesis. Theorizing that humans should seek the most energy-concentrated (i.e., the most natural) source of protein and calories, Bucky concluded that he should eat the meat of animals that eat plants.

By applying the unique idea of "energy accounting" to his weight problem, Bucky lost sixty pounds and greatly increased his energy. He continued to eat a low-carbohydrate diet for the rest of his life (he died at age eighty-eight).

All of the personalities discussed in this chapter can be understood as adherents to one of two philosophies of the human body: the thermodynamic view and the chaotic view. The thermodynamic view of the body sees a machine with parts to be balanced and manipulated. Thermodynamic nutritionists strive to create healthy, fit bodies by balancing caloric intake and output, by limiting dietary fat and cholesterol, by incorporating synthetic foods and supplements, and by prescribing strict exercise regimens. They treat the body like a steam engine that can be made to run on any kind of fuel with some simple adjustments. It's the calories-in/calories-out approach to human physiology and nutrition.

Thermodynamics can be used successfully to analyze a simple system, such as a steam engine, that has relatively few variables. The thermodynamic approach fails, however, when it is applied to a highly complex system, such as the human body, composed of large numbers of variables. In a system of great complexity, small changes in variables can produce drastically disproportionate and seemingly random results. In other words, you don't necessarily get out in proportion to what you put in—for our purposes, calories in don't equal calories out.

Consider what scientists call the Butterfly Effect: A butterfly flapping its wings in Africa can cause a hurricane in the Caribbean, because of the interaction of the components of planetary weather patterns. While the Butterfly Effect is an exaggerated scenario, it illustrates the fact that small changes in a system's variables (in this case, the components of global weather patterns) can produce results (a hurricane) that are unpredictable and disproportionate to the amount of energy expended (a butterfly flapping its wings). Small changes can have systemwide (global) implications.

Scientists in the 1970s noticed, however, that such seemingly random results in the evolution of a complex system actually display predictable patterns. These patterns are predictable as long as the original relationship between the system's original variables remains the same. The predictability of seemingly random change is now referred to as *chaos*. The study of chaotic systems is called *chaos theory*. Chaotic change is displayed in many of the forms that we see in nature, such as snowflakes and even the shapes of plant and animal life. Such forms are called *fractals*.

Fractal shaping is the reason that we can recognize snowflakes as snowflakes even though no single snowflake is shaped like any other. The same can be said of plants and animals of the same species regardless of their conditions of growth. Only when we introduce new variables—i.e., variables not part of a system's natural conditions—will results of a fractal shaping process become random and unpredictable, rendering the final shape unrecognizable. For example, by adding chemicals to water we can produce snowflakes that don't have six sides. And by exposing a healthy, pregnant mammal to high levels of radiation, we can produce offspring with severe physical abnormalities.

Stressing the body's "sensitive dependence on initial conditions" (see Gleick in Bibliography), chaos theory sees the human body as a highly complex, biological organism—not as an industrial machine that works according to a calories-in/calories-out model. You can never know or account for all the variables involved in the functioning of a system as complex as the human body. So a chaotic nutrition and fitness program doesn't add new variables to the equation. It won't try to reduce body fat by limiting dietary fat or to correct a vitamin deficiency by adding supplements. Instead, a chaotic approach stresses the removal of variables (agricultural diet, sedentary lifestyle) that aren't a part of the body's "initial conditions"—naked with a sharp stick on the African savanna.

But with all the dietary advice given throughout history, as well as the twentieth-century tidal wave of health research, how do we know which philosophy to follow? Whose science, whose research should we believe? Perhaps we need a new beginning. . . .

CHAPTER TWO

How a Stone Age Diet
Saved My Life

I have never been a fat person. I have weighed as much as twenty pounds more than my current weight, but even then I was considered thin. *NeanderThin* is not a result of trying to reduce my weight. *NeanderThin* is the result of my having other diseases that have the same causes as obesity.

More than twenty years ago, while a junior in college, I began to have problems with my joints. I frequently experienced sharp pains in my knees and other joints without traumatic injuries to explain the pain. After a trip to a doctor and several tests, I was informed that I had rheumatoid arthritis. I was told that it was an immune system disease and that both the cause and an effective treatment were unknown. The doctor suggested that I take lots of aspirin and use a cane when the pain became oppressive. He also told me that my condition would worsen in time, and his prediction proved to be painfully accurate.

A dozen years later—still taking lots of aspirin daily and walking with a cane—my career in computers was deteriorating along with my health. My energy seemed to diminish from year to year, a condition that I attributed to the arthritis. I began to experience severe headaches, tingling in my extremities, frequent urination, and constant thirst. My energy level was such that I could only work part-time, and I needed frequent naps.

My bad health was obviously destroying my life, so I sought medical advice once again. After consulting with several doctors, I was diagnosed as a diabetic and was told that I would probably require insulin injections for the rest of my life. Being only thirty-four years old at the time, this seemed to me a long and terrible prospect. I was also told that diabetes was an immune system disorder whose cause and cure were unknown.

Needless to say I was very disappointed with both my health problems and the medical community's inability to deal with them. I decided that I needed to know more about my condition in order to make my life productive once again. To that end I began my own research project at the public library. I studied the physiology of my conditions, as well as the history of the diseases and their treatments.

From my studies several things became clear: Both rheumatoid arthritis and diabetes are autoimmune system diseases in which the body uses its own defenses to attack itself. Both diseases also occur only within agricultural (civilized) communities. The more recently a population became agricultural, the more likely its members were to become diabetic. People like the Inuit and native North Americans, who were unlikely to have diabetes when eating their traditional diets, have the highest diabetes rates in the world (up to 80 percent of their population) when given the agricultural foods of civilization. From skeletal remains it has also been shown that arthritis followed corn as it made its way from Mexico to the rest of the world. Because my diseases were apparently diet-related, I decided I would modify my diet to emulate that of hunter-gatherers (preagricultural or Paleolithic peoples).

Eating a Natural Diet

My definition of nature is *the absence of technology*. Technology-dependent foods would never be ingested by a human being in nature. I determined, therefore, to eat only those foods that would be available to me if I were naked of all technology save that of a convenient sharp stick or stone.

Armed only with the sharp stick of my criterion, I headed for the supermarket. Before putting anything into my shopping cart, I thought carefully: Would this food be edible if I happened upon it as it grows in the wild and I had no technology or tools to make it edible?

During this experiment with a natural diet, I carefully tested my blood glucose to see if any improvement occurred. Expecting only modest results, I was astounded by what actually happened. My blood sugar levels returned to normal almost immediately and remained constant throughout the day. Every day it seemed I had more energy. I slept less than eight hours per day, whereas I had previously required at least ten. Although I lost a few pounds, I seemed to be getting bigger as my muscles became larger and more toned without special exercise. After a few weeks my joints stopped hurting almost completely. Even my ability to think and concentrate seemed to improve. Needless to say, my mood and overall attitude toward life changed for the better as well.

My curiosity was also piqued. Was I the only one to discover this miracle cure? I decided to use some of my newfound energy at the library to find out.

I began to look for similar diets in the medical library. It didn't take long to discover that the same diet was first prescribed to cure diabetes in the 1790s. Because the selection of foods was limited at the local market in that time period, the diet was very expensive and was thought to be impractical. Why it worked was not understood.

A very similar diet was found to be useful in the treatment of juvenile epilepsy beginning around the turn of the twentieth century. By replacing complex carbohydrates with fat—i.e., by having epileptics adopt a ketogenic diet—great improvements and even cures took place. The ketogenic diet was thought, however, to be impractical and even distasteful and was used only by a few hospitals (most notably Johns Hopkins) as a last resort. Why it worked was never successfully investigated, and it is only recently that many forms of epilepsy have been found to be immune system disorders. Dr. Robert C. Atkins popularized another variation of this diet beginning in the 1970s. Millions of people bought his book to lose weight and were successful. Dr. Irwin Stillman (the Stillman Water Diet) promoted an even stricter form. As these diets eliminate large amounts of alien proteins and result in weight loss, could that mean that obesity is also an immune system disorder? To answer this question we must look at what the immune system is designed to do as well as at the known immune system diseases and the characteristics that they share.

Understanding the Immune System

The purpose of the immune system is to protect the body from pathogens and parasites that are constantly attacking it. These attackers seek to rob the body of its food and energy and must be overcome in order to ensure survival. They include viruses, bacteria, germs, fungi, worms, insects, and other types of living things. Because of the number and diversity of attackers, the immune system must have a large number of defensive strategies. As most of these strategies are lethal to the targeted invader, great care must be taken in identifying them as alien and not part of the defending host's body—or its normal diet.

The immune system detects the presence of invaders by their alien protein structures: These are recognized as being different from the thousands of unique proteins that make up the body itself, its diet, and beneficial creatures such as the intestinal bacteria. When alien proteins are detected, the body can mount any of a number of defensive and offensive responses. Defensive responses include raising body temperature to render the body inhospitable to invaders (fever) or swelling to dilute any toxins that may be present (inflammation). Offensive responses include providing antibodies that signal white blood cells to attack alien proteins directly. The body may also try to expel the invaders mechanically through frequent defecation (in Latin, *dia-rea*) or frequent urination (in Latin, *dia-betis*).

With all the possible attackers and defenses, a large portion of the body's genetic makeup is the immune system. Indeed, the genetic diversity made possible by sexual reproduction allows a species as a whole to have many more possible immune responses than a single member of that species can possess. In a world in which attackers are numerous and constantly changing through mutation, this highly complex and adaptable defense system is vital for survival.

Some alien proteins, however, cause the immune system to attack the body itself, resulting in any one of the plethora of immune system diseases which abound in modern civilization. These proteins are introduced into the body through the consumption of unnatural foods that would not be available in a natural environment

Diseases of the immune system include arthritis, diabetes, allergies, colitis, Crohn's disease, multiple sclerosis, Alzheimer's, endometriosis, many forms of cancer, lupus, and most arterial diseases (heart attacks and strokes). The overwhelming majority (95 percent) of people in developed countries will die of immune system–related diseases. By contrast, these types of disorders are very rare in wild animals, even when one accounts for natural selection (predators and parasites) removing disabled individuals from their numbers. Among domesticated animals, however, which are fed diets far removed from their natural fare (e.g., American dogs who are fed cornmeal almost exclusively—inedible to their canine ancestors), immune system disorders are again very common. Other diseases that are not traditionally thought of as immune system disorders, such as epilepsy, tooth decay, myopia, appendicitis, mental illness, attention deficit disorder, chronic fatigue syndrome, acne, and emphysema, are also rare in nature.

For this reason, what we call immune system disorders were first grouped together as "diseases of civilization" by the French doctor Stanislas Tanchou in 1843. His monumental paper on this observation led to a one-hundred-year search for "civilized" disorders among primitive peoples by missionaries, whaling ship doctors, and explorers who had contact with these vanishing cultures. It was noted that, although the native population might be wiped out by infectious disease (smallpox, measles, mumps, etc.) at the outset of their contact with civilization, what we know as chronic immune system diseases were unknown to them. Only when the natives were introduced to the civilized foods did the "diseases of civilization" appear in their populations—in direct proportion to the degree of exposure.

As with allergies, other immune system diseases seem to exhibit a threshold of response. That is, until a certain level of exposure is achieved there is seemingly no reaction. You can be exposed to a specific allergen for years with no noticeable reaction and then suddenly develop symptoms. For instance, a tiny amount of pollen may trigger a hay fever attack if the immune system is already stressed by other allergies that, by themselves, cause no response. All immune system diseases seem to appear suddenly even though the alien proteins that cause them may have been present for years. This type of delayed reaction is necessary to prevent the body from responding to alien proteins that may be transitory or unable to survive in the environment found within the body for very long. By waiting until a threshold level is attained, the body avoids undue stress and conserves energy.

Another characteristic of immune system disorders is that not all people get them when exposed to the same alien proteins. The tendency to respond to a specific protein with an immune system disorder seems to be hereditary. As everyone's immune system is different and the DNA coding for the immune system comprises a large portion of the genetic code that one inherits from each parent, humans as a species can carry many more immunities to pathologies and parasites than any single human's DNA could carry. This ensures that some individuals in a population may survive any new parasite, pathogen, or plague.

All of these immune system disorder traits are shared by obesity, a condition virtually unknown among wild animals. Obesity often manifests as a threshold phenomenon—i.e., without changing diet or exercise patterns, a person may become obese. Moreover, no matter what the diet, not all people will become obese. There also seems to be a causal link between obesity and heredity. If your parents are disposed to carry excess body fat, odds are you are also.

Looking at people in many parts the world, one is amazed by the number of overweight individuals. These include both young and old and seem to be present in significant numbers in most places in which people are not facing severe famine.

Many people seek to lose excess body fat by reducing the amount of energy available to their bodies through a regimen of caloric restriction or exercise or both. These simple solutions almost never work. The top diet programs all share a very high failure rate. Even people who work out for a living (construction workers, longshoremen, warehouse workers, etc.) are prone to be overweight. Just look at the defensive and offensive lines of many football teams.

Caloric Restriction Is Not the Answer

Recent studies have also pointed out the contradictions inherent in attempting weight loss through caloric restriction. Poor people, who are most likely to perform manual labor and have little to spend on enticing foods, have the highest obesity rates. The Harvard Nutrition Study showed that overweight people actually eat significantly less than lean persons do. Involving 115,000 nurses who kept food diaries for twenty years, the Harvard Nutrition Study is regarded as the largest, most accurate nutrition survey ever conducted. Its results mirror studies performed on the efficacy of low-calorie diets funded by the Federal Trade Commission.

The FTC found that less than 5 percent of people who enrolled in low-calorie diet programs experienced long-term weight loss. A similar percentage of people on such programs develop eating disorders such as anorexia and bulimia, making the prognosis for weight loss through low-calorie eating less than encouraging. Using the evidence of their studies, the FTC won lawsuits against all of the major low-calorie weight loss programs. The defendants subsequently began adding disclaimers to their advertisements, stressing the importance of exercise and diet drugs. The results of these changes to their programs have yet to be determined by scientific study, except for the side effects of the drugs involved (most notably, Phen-Fen and Ma Huang).

Our current obsession with low-fat diets is also contradicted by many large-scale studies. In one such study at Texas Woman's College (now Texas Women's University) in the 1950s, researchers showed that of three experimental diets, the highest in fat produced greater weight loss than the moderate and low-fat diets also employed. A recent study published in the *Journal of the American Medical Association* (see Garg in Bibliography) showed that LDL ("bad") cholesterol levels actually rose appreciably (average 24 percent) on a low-fat diet among insulin-resistant individuals (the vast majority of whom are overweight). Triglycerides also rose by 25 percent. These findings prompted the doctors involved in the study to discontinue their research to avoid harming the study's subjects and to allow the doctors to rethink the viability of a low-fat diet for those most at risk for heart disease.

Obesity is very rare in nature. Unlike many of the animals we see in zoos, overweight wild animals are virtually unknown. This seems to be the case even when unlimited amounts of food are available. The reasons for this are apparent when we look at the harsh realities of nature. An overweight animal would be slower and more prone to be eaten by predators. An overweight predator would be less successful in catching its prey. Any obese animal would be more prone to disease. All of these factors would mean fewer offspring and a lessening of that species' chances for survival.

Obviously, obesity puts an animal on the losing side of the natural selection process. Why then should it be so common in humans, domesticated animals, and even the wild animals kept by man in zoos? The answer is found by analyzing the technologies of civilization that separate the artificial world of man from the natural environment.

An Evolutionary Approach to Health and Weight Loss

The main theme of *NeanderThin* is that eating foods made edible by civilized technologies is the root cause of numerous diseases in both civilized man and his domesticated animals—diseases that are rarely found under more natural conditions. Indeed, if we look at the skeletal remains of man prior to 10,000 years ago—before the technological innovation of the Neolithic (Agricultural) Revolution—we find no evidence of obesity and very little evidence of the plethora of other immune system diseases that are so common today.

When we examine the remains of humans immediately following the Neolithic Revolution, we see at once evidence of the obesity and diseases common in the modern world. Our Neolithic ancestors' transition from hunting and gathering to farming resulted in a substantial decrease in life span and a decrease of several inches in average height (see Harris in Bibliography). Paleoanthropologists and archaeologists find that these characteristics combine to form a convenient yardstick in determining the technology level of the ancient people being studied—the more diseased the population, the greater the technological sophistication of its culture.

As we are talking about ancient people, the technologies involved are not those we commonly think of in this world of computers and rockets to the moon, but rather the simple practices of cooking and agriculture used by all people today and in the historic past. Even the most primitive methods of cooking and agriculture have broad implications concerning what humans eat and, consequently, our overall health.

This book is not meant to be an indictment of technology. Since about 1850, when we started living longer and growing taller (at least in industrial societies), technology has extended and improved our lives dramatically in many ways. Mathematically, these benefits do not correlate with the advancements in medical science or improvements in general hygiene. Modern advances in human health correlate very closely with the rate at which new transportation methods such as railroads, steamboats, cars, and airplanes improved our diets. Following the NeanderThin diet plan would have been difficult only fifty years ago and nearly impossible a hundred years ago.

Sharpen Your Sticks and Get Ready to Eat

Just as if we were trying to formulate the ideal diet for a newly discovered zoo animal, we will look at man, his unique physical attributes and ancestral environment, to determine his ideal natural diet: a diet that will satisfy our need for food without compromising our health or waistlines; *more important, a diet that will allow us to eat as much food as we need to feel satisfied and full.*

No special foods will be required for this diet. All you need are foods that you can get from almost any supermarket. At no time will you count calories or the size of portions on your plate. Most people following the NeanderThin program find that food preparation is greatly simplified.

It sounds very easy, but it's not. Most overweight people will have to permanently give up many of their favorite foods. Fortunately, the cravings for these foods will pass very quickly for those who commit themselves to the program 100 percent from the very beginning. Any sacrifice will be compensated for by the ability to eat as much as you want, whenever you want. Many people find they are eating more food than ever before and still losing weight.

You can get a general idea of how to follow the NeanderThin diet by skimming through the book. But if you read the entire book, you will have a solid understanding as to why agricultural, civilized foods are detrimental to your health and weight. Your understanding will motivate you to stay with this nutrition plan until it becomes part of your lifestyle. For the majority (at least 99.5 percent) of human history, it was the only diet we knew.

CHAPTER THREE

How Our Place in the Food Chain Determines Our Diet

In order to understand the makeup of our natural diet, it is first necessary to understand what kind of animal we are. We must compare ourselves to other creatures and determine how our similarities, as well as our unique features, contribute to our success within the environment we were designed to inhabit.

Man is classified by science as a primate. The order *Primata* is believed to have evolved from the order *Insectivora* (insect-eating mammals). The order *Primata* includes many other species of animals such as lemurs, monkeys, and apes, which in numerous respects closely resemble humans. We share many family traits including an opposable thumb, binocular vision, and (with the possible exception of one species of monkey) an omnivorous diet. More than 95 percent of primates have a single-chambered stomach incapable of digesting most complex carbohydrates as they occur in nature (in the absence of technology). Of the 200 species of primates, only the Colobus and Langur monkeys (about ten species) have a multichambered stomach and are, thus, capable of digesting grains and other complex carbohydrates in their natural, raw form.

An omnivorous diet includes both animal and vegetable foods. The ratio of meats to vegetable matter varies greatly between individual species of primates. The tree shrew subsists almost entirely on insects while other primates, such as the gorilla, get 90 percent of their food from fruits and vegetables. All are, however, designed by nature to maximize the food resources available in their environmental niche. Most primates are found within the tropical forest or at its edges. The forest provides a wide variety of fruits, vegetables, insects, and small game that compose the diet of arboreal primates.

The earliest remains of hominids are found on the African savanna. To see how this primeval grassland appeared, all we need to do is look at any lawn or golf course. Indeed, anthropologists explain our compulsion to install lawns no matter where we find ourselves as a need to re-create the environment for which we were designed and in which we, therefore, feel most comfortable.

Within this savanna environment, man is the only primate (although baboons can be found on its edges). It is very different from the environment favored by most primates. There are few of the trees whose fruit and leaves provide the bulk of food for the creatures of the forest. Life on the savanna is dominated by grasses, grass-eating animals called herbivores, and the carnivores and omnivores that, in turn, prey upon these herbivores.

In the process of adapting to a grassland habitat, the evolving hominid developed several physical characteristics unique in the animal kingdom. These adaptations are what separate us from our primate relatives and help to define our specific niche in the ecological system.

What Makes Humans Unique

Our unique characteristics include a large lopsided brain, bipedalism, eye dominance (resulting in handedness), a lack of fur, and a unique variety of sweat glands. None of these physical traits (except bipedalism in some bird species) is found in other animals. By determining the evolutionary advantages made possible by these traits, we will develop a better picture of the niche man was created to inhabit.

In nature, brain capacity is related to the types of activities the associated creature engages in most frequently. Predators consistently have proportionately larger brains than herbivores of the same size because the activity of hunting requires more cognitive functions than simply eating the next leaf. The largest brains of all are usually found in omnivores. Omnivores must eat a much wider range of plant and animal foods to survive and must, therefore, have a greater capacity to develop and remember the strategies needed to obtain these foods.

Man, with his proportionately largest of all brains, is capable of obtaining and eating the largest number of other species of plants and animals of any known creature. This trait is invaluable in the savanna where no single group of species produces enough food to sustain humans year round. It also allows humans to outsmart creatures who are faster, bigger, or have better senses than we do, and to add these species to our available food resources.

One theory concerning hominid brain size postulates that our brains had to increase in size in response to the stress placed on our intellects by our Paleolithic social environment. The success of the hunting and gathering lifestyle requires cooperation among group members. The interplay that is seen in such interactions as trading, sharing, sexual pairing, and communal child rearing required that humans develop a sophisticated, if only intuitive, awareness of social morality. The ability to create and maintain strong group relationships is necessary in any species that relies on hunting for the main part of its diet. Indeed, humans share the moral values of altruism and compassion with other species of carnivorous pack animals. Herbivores, which have proportionately small brains, don't display such sophisticated moral behavior.

A large brain does have disadvantages. It burns a lot of fuel. And, because of our large brain size, humans are physically less developed at birth than other animals. As a result our infants require a much longer maturation period than other similar, but smaller-brained, apes and monkeys.

The archaeological record confirms that hominid brain size increased in concert with the developing sophistication of stone tools, which allowed for more efficient hunting of large, calorie-rich game. Because the larger hominid brain required more energy, the body evolved to derive greater amounts of energy from food even as the digestive system became smaller in relation to both brain size and total body size. This "expensive tissue hypothesis" (see Aiello in Bibliography) explains why the evolving hominid could no longer survive on the low-energy-value foods favored by the other smaller-brained, but larger-gutted, great apes.

Understanding the Digestive System

The disproportionately small human gut is unique among primates. Like other primates our food is absorbed through both a small and large intestine. The small intestine absorbs food directly through the action of digestive enzymes. In the large intestine bacteria continue the digestive process, breaking down complex carbohydrates, such as fiber and starch, into simple carbohydrates that can be absorbed by the walls of the large intestine for assimilation by the body.

The size ratio of small to large intestine (gut ratio) varies considerably from one species to another. Compared to other primates, humans have a shrunken large intestine and colon. Our relatively small lower gastrointestinal tract inhibits our ability to extract nutrients from calorically sparse foods (leaves, stems, shoots, bark, etc.), making us more dependent on calorically dense foods such as meat, fruit, and nuts. The shrinking of the hominid colon occurred in a short period of evolutionary time (only a few million years) as is evidenced by the failure of the lymph node attached to the colon to shrink along with the human colon. This lymph node is called the appendix.

Only two other creatures on earth have an appendix: the rabbit and the wombat. Both of these creatures eat calorically sparse foods but have evolved the habit of passing their food through their digestive tracts twice—i.e., they eat their feces. This adaptation allows them to derive extra nutrients from their food similar to the manner in which ruminants (cows, goats, sheep, etc.) regurgitate their cud to pass it through their digestive systems a second time. Because we humans have short large intestines and digest our food only once, it is necessary for us to eat calorie-rich foods to meet our nutritional requirements.

In comparing the gut ratio of humans to other primates, the closest ratios are found in Capuchin monkeys and swamp baboons, both of which eat more meat than any other primates (except humans). These two species also have hands that are the most dexterous and human-like of all lower primates. But even their gut ratios are far different from ours. The human gut ratio is most comparable to carnivores, particularly the wolf. Anthropologists have long postulated that the similarities in the diets of wolves/dogs and humans played a pivotal role in their becoming our first domestic animals.

Other Advantages to Being Human

Bipedalism, or walking on two legs, is found only in humans and flightless birds such as the ostrich. Both humans and ostriches realize several important advantages through this mode of locomotion. The first is maximum eye height for body size, resulting in a wide range of vision across the broad plains of the savanna they both inhabited. This trait is very useful whether you are looking for food or avoiding predators. The second advantage is the energy efficiency of bipedal locomotion first exploited by the dinosaurs more than 100

EAT RIGHT FOR YOUR GUT TYPE

The connection between the digestive tract and nutrition was first noted in 1888 by Dr. James Salisbury in his book *The Relation of Alimentation and Disease*. Dr. Salisbury, for whom the famous chopped steak is named, recommended a diet composed of one part vegetables and fruits and two parts meat. His book created a sensation among those wishing to lose weight. His diet also increased demand for the meat of tough Texas longhorn cattle.

In his 1975 book entitled *The Stone Age Diet*, Dr. Walter L. Voegtlin (see Bibliography), a leading gastroenterologist of his day, compared the human digestive tract to that of the dog using a chart originally from Salisbury's book. His "Type-A diet" for patients with serious digestive ailments was even more restrictive than Salisbury's, requiring that the few vegetables be boiled and drained before eaten. He permitted those persons who were "only obese" a few more raw vegetables. Dr. Voegtlin's "maintenance diet" included one serving of bread per day.

million years ago. Whether you are a *Tyrannosaurus rex,* a roadrunner, or a human, this energy efficiency gives you a tremendous advantage over your four-legged prey. As a human, when walking or running your hands are free to use a weapon, which, if thrown while moving, greatly increases the weapon's velocity (some baseball players throw rock-size balls over 100 miles per hour). Bipedalism also allows us to use our hands to carry food over large distances more efficiently than other primates. This long-distance carrying ability allows us (through sharing) a highly efficient division of labor in our hunting and gathering efforts.

With proper conditioning and training, almost any able-bodied human can run a marathon. Indeed only one other predator can keep up with a man over long distances—our traditional hunting partner, the dog. But dogs can achieve such endurance only under cool weather conditions. In warmer climates, man's endurance easily surpasses that of the dog or any other predator. The physical endurance humans achieve is not limited by climate because of our lack of fur and our unique cooling system.

Our ancestral home, the equatorial African savanna, has a very warm climate year round. During the heat of the midday sun, almost all animal activity comes to a halt. Predators hunt during dawn and dusk or at night. Grazing animals move as little as possible in the heat of the midday and seek the few shade trees and wallow holes that are available. Only man is capable of sustained physical activity in all but the very hottest hours of the day. This advantage opens a window of opportunity for hunting when competition from other predators is scant and prey animals are sluggish.

Human sweat is formulated to evaporate very quickly when compared to the sweat of other mammals. We are also capable of sweating a much greater volume of liquid than other creatures. Our bare skin exposes this efficient coolant directly to the wind and sun, aiding the evaporation process. The hair on our heads keeps the hot rays of the sun off our heads where we are most prone to overheating. This efficient cooling system allows humans strenuous levels of activity under high temperature conditions that would quickly cause other animals extreme distress.

Because man also has his primate opposable thumb and his hands are free when walking, as stated previously, he can carry objects or food over large distances. This is one of man's most important traits, as it allows him to not only use tools as other apes do but also to carry these tools from place to place and use them for multiple purposes. The ability to carry food also helps overcome the disadvantage of a slowly maturing infant by enabling others to help in gathering food for both mother and child.

The hand is our principal eating utensil, and the shape of the human hand tells us much about our natural diet. In nature, most primate hands are considerably different from ours. Most primate thumbs are far less opposable than the human thumb. Several arboreal primates that eat mostly fruit lack thumbs altogether. The hands of Capuchin monkeys and baboons, both of which eat the most meat of any nonhominid primates, resemble human hands more than any other primate species. (The ability to grab your food is very important when your food is trying to escape.)

Even before hominid brains developed the great size evident in modern humans, they developed a unique shape. All hominid brains exhibit longitudinal asymmetry (lopsidedness). Eye dominance, produced by the unique shape of our brain, produced handedness, which—when combined with our carrying ability—resulted in a new skill unparalleled in any other life form: the ability to throw an object with accuracy. This ability is what has allowed humans to become the most efficient hunters on earth. It has given us the ability to hunt not only small game as monkeys and other apes do, but also to hunt animals much larger and/or faster than we are. A single human with a sharp stick can kill any other creature on earth—a claim a Bengal tiger would envy.

Using these gifts of evolution, humans developed one of the most diverse diets known in the animal world. A wide variety of fruits, vegetables, nuts, and berries could easily be gathered or dug from the ground with simple tools and eaten without further processing. Almost any animal food, including small and large game, could be hunted successfully. These foods could be brought back to a central location to be shared with all members of the group. When foraging for vegetable foods or hunting became difficult because of the season or overconsumption, humans could easily move themselves and their few tools to a new location without need of domestic draft animals.

Hominids lived this way for over 2 million years. Today we call this lifestyle hunter-gathering. We were so successful at it that humans were able to expand beyond their original environment to virtually all parts of the world. The period of time when humans were hunter-gatherers is known as the Paleolithic Era. This era lasted until about 10,000 years ago when the new technologies of agriculture were ushered in during the period known as the Neolithic Era. By examining the lifestyle (see Appendix A for in-depth information) of Paleolithic man and his changing environment, we can come to a better understanding of how the transition to agriculture changed our lives and health.

CHAPTER FOUR

How We Lived and Ate Before Agriculture

Although hunter-gathering has largely disappeared as a lifestyle in today's world, much is known about how hunter-gatherers lived and ate. By examining the fossil remains of Paleolithic humans (bones, feces, and artifacts) and by studying the lives of people such as the African Bushmen and Arctic Inuit (Eskimo), who persisted in hunter-gathering into the twentieth century, scientists have a clear picture of how these people lived and died.

Hunter-gatherers lived quite well compared to the way they are often portrayed in contemporary works of fiction. In many ways they enjoyed considerably better conditions than the Neolithic and modern people who followed them.

The search for food among hunter-gatherers has often been thought of as a long and laborious process by those of us who are used to the convenience of supermarkets. Studies of contemporary hunter-gatherers, dispell this myth conclusively. Among hunter-gatherers living in the harshest desert and Arctic conditions, it has been found that they work less than 3 hours per day. These hours not only include the time necessary to obtain and prepare food but also the time to provide housing and clothing.

Human physical traits, as well as the sheer number of food

sources available in nature, explain the ease by which hunter-gatherers obtain food. Although modern man gets 90 percent of his calories from just twenty species of plants and animals, a typical Paleolithic hunter-gatherer got his nutrition from over a hundred species. All of these sources were edible raw and required little processing. Only very recently have an affluent minority of people gained access to a similar variety of foods. The development of modern transportation systems, accompanied by multicultural demand in urban centers created by large-scale immigration, has made possible the large variety of foods available in wealthy countries.

Famine is virtually unknown among hunter-gatherers. Drought serves only to make game easier to obtain as the weakened animals cluster at the few remaining water holes. If these dried up, people would simply move to a new area. As man was used to seasonal migrations to follow the game herds and the fruiting of plants, relocation would cause no unusual hardship.

With all of these food sources available, man did not hesitate to eat his fill. Recent studies of contemporary hunter-gatherers have shown that they ate considerably more food every day than the average American. As their food-gathering and other activities burned fewer calories than a leisurely round of golf, we would expect these people to be quite heavy. This is not the case.

Lean, Thin, and Healthy

These same studies have shown hunter-gatherers to have the lowest fat to total body weight ratio of any people on earth. Hunter-gatherers also show amazing physical fitness and muscle tone when compared to similar agricultural people who work longer and harder every day in the course of their farming activities.

The general health of Paleolithic hunter-gatherers was also excellent. The average life expectancy of a Paleolithic hunter-gatherer was approximately 33 years for men and 28 years for women (see Harris's *Cannibals and Kings* in Bibliography). Most evidence of early death from this period indicates that the principal causes were infectious disease, trauma, and the perils of childbirth. A hunter-gatherer who survived these hazards could expect to live as long as we do today. Moreover, the remains of those who did survive into middle age showed few signs of the chronic tooth decay, osteoporosis, obesity, diabetes, cancer, heart disease, and arthritis that plague our older population.

The health of contemporary hunter-gatherers has also been studied extensively. Perhaps the most in-depth survey ever done was performed in the early twentieth century by a dentist, Weston Price, who investigated the origins and causes of tooth decay. In his book *Nutrition and Physical Degeneration,* he documented the almost complete absence of degenerative diseases in the most primitive of cultures. In cooperation with Frances Pottenger, M.D., who researched the effects of cooking on the nutritional value of foods, Price created the Price Pottenger Nutrition Foundation. To this day the foundation continues to research the health of modern hunter-gatherers.

Professor Loren Cordain of Colorado State University has amassed a library of over 15,000 references in the scientific literature concerning Paleolithic health and nutrition. Included in Dr. Cordain's library are several studies of contemporary Australian aborigines. One such study (see O'Dea in Bibliography) highlights the detrimental effects of changing their traditional hunter-gatherer diet to a civilized diet. Conversely, when the aborigines return to the bush and their native diet, their health improves drastically.

Man's "New" Best Friend

During the prehistoric period known as the Pleistocene, severe climatic changes required mankind to alter his lifestyle. The expansion and contraction of the polar ice fields due to several Ice Ages resulted in an increase in the area of the earth covered by grasslands. In adapting to these much cooler, temperate grasslands, man invented methods of coping with lower temperatures not encountered in his original tropical range. These adaptations included new types of clothing and the use of fire to stay warm.

As man's range extended into this new temperate grassland, he encountered many types of animals that thrived in this environment. Along with mammoths, mastodons, woolly rhinoceroses, and giant ground sloths, there was an animal that closely resembled man in diet and pack behavior. This creature was the wolf. Because a wolf diet is almost identical to that of humans, wolves followed human tribes to eat their leftovers, just as humans would often chase a wolf pack from a kill to steal its meat. Only those wolves and humans that tolerated the other species would benefit from this symbiotic relationship.

In a recent experiment at a Siberian fox farm, it was found that foxes bred for tameness (tolerance of another species) changed dramatically in both behavior and physical form after only 15 generations. Their skulls became shorter, their tails curled, their coats developed distinctive patches of color, and they began to bark. In short, they became dogs. These doglike traits are normal in juvenile canines but are absent in mature foxes and wolves. The process of mutation that leads to a retention of juvenile traits into maturity is called *neoteny*. Under laboratory conditions this transformation took less than 20 years (see Budiansky in Bibliography).

Under field conditions the selection process leading to the neotenization of wolves was much subtler. The near-term result was only a slight survival advantage for those wolves and humans who learned to coexist and cooperate. Therefore, the transformation of wolves to dogs took many thousands of years. The change is documented not so much by the physical remains of early dogs—which were little more than tame wolves—but, rather, by man's use of new hunting tools made practical by a new hunting partnership with dogs.

Hunting methods can often be inferred from the tools used. To hunt any large game animal, you must first bring it within the range of your weapon. When you are hunting with other humans, you surround your prey and hold it within a very close range. Heavy rocks and stout spears are best under these circumstances. This is a very dangerous method of hunting, as evidenced by the injury patterns in the remains of early hunters. These rodeo-style injuries are unavoidable when attacking animals many times the size of the hunter.

When dogs were employed to hold prey animals within weapons' range, hunters could use long-range weapons (slings, arrows, light spears with throwing sticks, etc.) from a much safer distance. Without the assistance of dogs, long-range projectile weapons are much less efficient. Although they can be used in stalking or ambushing large game (as in modern bow hunting), after the first shot the animal will bolt. Only if the game is held at bay will it not run, allowing for follow-up shots. To hit a moving target or a vital area of a stationary target is very difficult, even with a modern compound bow or crossbow. To bring down very large animals (mammoths, wooly rhinoceroses) with a single arrow or a light throwing spear is nearly impossible.

Short-range use of long-range projectile weapons can be a liability for the hunter. To see why this is so, imagine shooting an arrow into a bear. As hazardous as this can be at a distance of 50 feet, at less than 10 feet the hunter is in greater danger than the bear. A lighter spear or an arrow is practically useless when defending against the lethal charge of a bear or another large animal. At such close range a long, stout spear is a much safer choice of weapon. Only when accompanied by dogs could primitive humans safely and effectively hunt with long-range weapons.

Entering into this relationship with wolves was made easy by the manner in which wolves hunt. Wolves are highly efficient at chasing large prey animals to exhaustion and surrounding them. They are, however, inefficient killers. It is not uncommon for a wolf pack to hold a larger animal such as a moose at bay for several days before they manage to kill it. Humans coming upon such a scene would have made quick work of the frightened, wounded prey.

Whenever a species rapidly expands its geographic range, neotenized members of the species will enjoy a slight advantage in exploiting the resources of a new environment. It is more efficient for a creature to retain juvenile traits than to evolve completely new ones for survival in a new ecological niche. The wanderlust and curiosity that these members retain from their youth allow them to exploit food choices in new territory. Wolves and humans rapidly expanded their range due to the waxing and waning of Ice Ages, long before they entered into a symbiotic relationship.

Both species had previously begun the process of neoteny before joining forces. When wolves and humans entered into a relationship, this process was accelerated into what we now call domestication. Wolves were eventually transformed into more gracile (i.e., thinner) dogs and Neanderthals into Cro-Magnons (*Homo sapiens sapiens* or NeanderThins if you will). The resulting mixed packs of dogs and humans were able to take game that neither wolves nor men could take alone. Mankind and his canine partners spread across the world, hunting many large animals into extinction in a very short period of time.

Although new technologies (use of fire, new clothing) enabled man to expand his range dramatically, there were only slight changes in man's food-gathering and hunting traditions. Animals were now hunted for their fur as well as their meat. Meats could now be preserved by drying and smoking them in racks above the warming fire. These new techniques supplanted the process of sun drying meat to preserve it that had existed for millennia. The same types of plants that were edible raw continued to provide the vegetable component of our omnivorous diet.

Just before the end of the Paleolithic Era, the new use of fire, along with the neotenization of several other animal species (goats, sheep, cows), allowed man to eat many types of plants and animal products (dairy) that without technological intervention would not be edible by human beings. With the extinction of the Pleistocene megafauna, caused in part by the sudden appearance of the new super predator—man-dog packs—new food sources were needed. These new food sources would, with the Neolithic Revolution, become the staples of the modern diet. This revolution wouldn't be completed until the last hunter-gatherers were rendered virtually extinct in the twentieth century. The first casualty of this struggle was to be our health.

CHAPTER FIVE

The Agricultural Revolution

Evidence of abrupt change in the behavior and health of people in certain regions is seen in their remains dating from about 10,000 years ago. These changes were brought about by man's new reliance on technology-dependent foods for his sustenance.

About 12,000 years ago the last Ice Age ended, and our current interglacial period began. For the first time in over 100,000 years, the ice sheets retreated fully into the deep Arctic. Those areas in the temperate zone that had been lush grasslands—i.e., steppe-tundra—became dry savannas or, in some cases, deserts. With the regression of the ice sheets, sea levels rose, flooding many coastal areas that were formerly part of the steppe-tundra. This flooding disrupted animal migrations by eliminating land bridges.

In higher latitudes forests grew to extend over immense tracts of land that were once covered by ice. These forestlands could not sustain human populations at densities as high as those in the dry savannas and not even close to the densities of those populations in the disappearing steppe-tundra. As conditions in the temperate zone became warmer and drier, humans had to develop alternate food sources if they were to survive.

Man Learns to Cook

Fortunately, man had already domesticated fire. Using fire for warmth was an old practice. At the end of the Paleolithic Era, man learned to cook. Meat that was drying or thawing by the fire would become roasted on its surface and people soon began to enjoy this new taste. Some traditional raw vegetable foods were also found to taste better roasted when they were accidentally dropped into the fire.

Soon, plants that had never been eaten before were found to be edible when they were accidentally cooked. Seeds that were on the grasses close to the fire were found to have a new nutlike flavor and to be nutritionally satisfying. Soon grains were added to man's diet. Sometimes when fires were built over certain plants, the previously inedible roots would be found in the ashes to join the new menu as potatoes and yams. Likewise, the seedpods of certain shrubs became our beans and other legumes when their branches were used as fuel for the fire, and they were found to be tasty and filling when roasted.

These new foods never became very prominent in the late Paleolithic diet. Although they were easily stored for long periods of time, carrying them from place to place was impractical, as the hunter-gatherer bands moved to follow the seasonal migrations of the herds and the fruiting of plants.

Normally, when grass seeds become mature, they fall to the ground and become very difficult to harvest. A subtle, unconscious selection process began among plants made edible by cooking. Grass stems that never fully matured were preferred during harvest. Man would carry these, in turn, to the prime real estate next to the waterhole where he had set up his campsite and food preparation area.

Excess and waste grass seeds grew in man's highly fertilized dumpsites (i.e., latrines). When man returned to these sites in his seasonal wanderings to again gather the grasses, he found more readily harvested plants growing very close to his old campsite. Thus, through man's unconscious selection process over many generations of grasses, new types of plants emerged. We call them grains. Eventually, this juvenile trait of seed retention resulted in plants that could not propagate without seed separation from the stem (i.e., threshing) by man. These plants became totally dependent upon man in a new system of food production. Similarly, other unconscious selection processes based on taste, color, size, and harvestability led to other plants being incorporated into this new food production system we call agriculture.

The Invention of Agriculture

It was the invention of agriculture about 10,000 years ago that resulted in these new foods becoming the staples that they are in today's diet. By planting the seeds of these plants, man found that he could obtain large harvests. Large amounts of food could then be stored, dried, and consumed throughout the year. Because of the need to tend, harvest, and protect his crops, man largely abandoned his former seasonal wanderings and settled down into the first permanent settlements.

This need to preserve foods led to other technologies. Pottery vessels were invented about 6,000 years ago and were used to store the new staples. Soon pots were to join other inventions such as grinding stones and ovens in new cooking techniques such as boiling and baking. These implements further hindered man's ability to be nomadic by the sheer difficulty of transporting them without domesticated draft animals.

As the areas around permanent settlements quickly became depleted of game and wild vegetable foods, Neolithic settlers became more dependent on crops for the majority of their food.

These staples were supplemented by small amounts of meat and, for the first time, milk from domestic animals. The Neolithic diet had immediate effects on man's health. The skeletons of Neolithic farmers show the effects of poor nutrition. They died much younger (see Cohen in Bibliography), were shorter, and had many more cavities, as well as fewer teeth, than their immediate hunter-gatherer ancestors (see Harris's *Cannibals and Kings* in Bibliography). These same remains also show the first evidence of obesity in humans.

The tendency to put on weight was to have another effect on the living conditions of Neolithic peoples. In spite of a much shorter life span, population densities grew dramatically. As women must have a certain minimum percentage of body fat to ovulate, the tendency of agricultural people to become fat resulted in women becoming pregnant at an earlier age and becoming pregnant again much sooner after giving birth. Studies of contemporary female hunter-gatherers have shown them to reach first menstruation several years later than agricultural women. Hunter-gatherer women averaged four years between births versus eleven months for agricultural women. As it was no longer necessary to carry infants from place to place, the natural constraints on family size experienced by nomadic hunter-gatherers were no longer in effect.

Obviously, greater populations required larger crop yields for sustenance. Methods of agricultural intensification such as the plow and irrigation were soon invented to boost yields. As these more intensive methods accelerated the exhaustion of the topsoil and populations continued to grow, new lands for cultivation had to be found. The process of colonization continued until recent history, until the civilized world became agricultural, polluted, overpopulated, and overweight.

CHAPTER SIX

Why Agricultural Foods
Are Bad for You

We have seen how humans are designed to eat and how dietary patterns have been changed by agriculture. In order to eliminate the problems of the modern diet, we must return to the natural diet of our Paleolithic ancestors. The easiest way to accomplish this goal is to imagine oneself stripped of all technology except a sharp stick or rock and to eat only those foods that would be edible under these circumstances. When we look at foods in this light, it is very simple to distinguish between natural and technology-dependent foods.

Foods that require technological intervention (i.e., cooking and, in the case of milk, domestication) to be made edible include grains, beans, potatoes, milk, and sugar. All of these, when found in the wild in their original state, are impossible for us to eat. To eat in a Paleolithic manner, it is necessary to eliminate these foods from our diet completely.

Going Against the Grain

Grains include wheat, corn, rice, oats, barley, rye, and many other seeds of grasses imported from all over the world. Without milling and long cooking all are inedible to humans. When ground, raw grain becomes raw flour and fiber—just add water and you have papier-mâché, which if ingested will cause severe digestive problems in any primate (ask any elementary school teacher). Most grains are also mutants resulting from agricultural breeding practices and have no botanical equivalent in the wild. Most grains have even lost the ability to reproduce themselves without mechanical threshing by man to remove the grain from the stem.

Countless studies have shown that when people eat grains containing large amounts of cellulose fiber (as found in whole grains), which passes through the body undigested, risk of contracting cancer and heart disease is reduced in direct proportion to the amount of added fiber. Similar proportional reductions in risk are observed when fruit and vegetable consumption is increased at the expense of technology-dependent foods.

These observations have led many scientists to conclude that bran and chemicals found in fruits and vegetables (phytates, etc.) are panaceas for reducing cancer and heart disease risk. As a result, consumers have spent countless millions of dollars for supplements containing these "silver bullets."

Modern, statistically valid studies of cancer and heart disease rates among people eating a Paleolithic diet have never been performed. Such peoples became almost completely extinct prior to the development of scientific epidemiological research techniques. Anecdotal findings, such as those reported by Vilhjalmur Stefansson in his book *Cancer: Disease of Civilization,* imply a complete lack of such diseases in hunter-gather populations.

"From the corn fields, one of the most potent cancer-causing agents known to science is coursing into the nation's food supply" ("Corn-Crop Peril," *Wall Street Journal,* February 23, 1989). The 6,500-word article this quote is taken from refers to aflatoxin, a substance produced by asparilla rust (just one of several types of toxin-producing rusts that can infect any grain crop). This rust is a fungus that infects corn and other crops, such as peanuts, under certain conditions of heat and humidity. Aflatoxins have been linked to liver, pancreatic, and esophageal cancers in some of the laboratory animals tested.

In 1998, 62% of the Texas corn crop tested exceeded government-approved levels (20 parts per billion) of aflatoxin ("Texas Journal," *Wall Street Journal*, July 29, 1998) and was deemed unfit for human consumption. Some samples tested indicated levels as high as 1,000 parts per billion. Most of the rejected grain had aflatoxin levels of fewer than 300 parts per billion and was approved for sale as animal food.

The American dog population has considerably higher rates of cancer than humans in this country (ask your vet). Consider also that the most common ingredient in commercial dog foods is this cheap, contaminated corn. While the connection between canine cancer rates and corn consumption has not been adequately researched, many dog-food producers are preemptively replacing corn with rice in their formulations.

Grains are found in many more products than the expected breads and breakfast cereals, often being used as fillers or thickeners in other foods. Extracts from grains such as corn oil, corn syrup, maltose, and others are also used to add fat or sweetness to a wide variety of processed foods.

Spilling the Beans

Beans are defined as seeds of legume plants, but the term *bean* is often used in reference to berries and nuts that are inedible raw (e.g., coffee beans). Many beans are extremely toxic if consumed raw, such as limas and soy, while others can only be safely consumed raw for a few days during their immature state (e.g., green beans). Some, such as peas and peanuts, are not considered beans in our culture.

Toxic compounds called *alkaloids* are found in all species of legumes (see Stahl and McGee in Bibliography). These natural pesticides protect beans from the creatures that would eat them in the wild. Several of these toxic compounds are cyanogens such as cyanide. Wild lima beans exhibit a heavy concentration of cyanide. When boiling lima beans, cyanide gas—used by some states in criminal executions—is expelled.

Fava plants contain the toxins vicine, covicine, and isouramil. These toxins are ingested by eating the beans, pods, or other parts of the fava plant or by inhaling the plant's pollen. In persons deficient in the enzyme G6PD, fava toxins are not broken down upon digestion. The toxins inhibit red blood cells in their delivery of oxygen to the various tissues in the body, resulting in a condition called *favism*. Symptoms can range from headaches, dizziness, nausea, and yawning to vomiting, severe abdominal pain, and fever. The acute hemolytic anemia experienced in the most serious cases of favism is often fatal.

Almost all toxins from legume (bean and pea) plants are broken down by cooking. (Although victims of favism almost always contract the disease after eating cooked fava beans). Almost no evidence exists that eating cooked beans will harm humans (except perhaps socially because of flatulence). That cooking is required to eat beans is enough, however, to exclude them from a Paleolithic diet.

Extracts from beans also find wide use in processed foods. Soy proteins are often added as a meat substitute, and peanut oil is used as a cheap source of fat in many products.

The Problem with Potatoes

When the Inca conquered other peoples, the surrender ceremony consisted of making their new subjects eat potatoes. Because potatoes could feed many subjects on little land, their Inca overlords could take more resources as tribute. Later, the English used this same strategy in Ireland.

Most people are aware that there are poisons found in the eye of potatoes. Most, however, are unaware that these same toxins, primarily the alkaloids solanine and chaconine, are found in the entire potato. Wild potatoes, and those improperly stored, contain much higher levels of these compounds than do domestic, unspoiled potatoes, and consuming these raw can result in lethal dosages.

A staple diet of potatoes can lead to a severe vitamin A deficiency, a leading cause of blindness in children in many parts of the world. Because of the prevalence of fungal breakouts in cultivated potatoes, they must be treated with large amounts of fungicides. The Inca overcame this problem by inventing freeze-drying in the cold, dry climate of the Andes Mountains. Instant potatoes are produced by this method today.

It should be noted that the effects of a lifetime of regular exposure to tiny amounts of the aforementioned toxins, fungus, and fungicides are largely unknown. Since our Paleolithic ancestors ate potatoes rarely if ever, all varieties of potatoes are excluded from the NeanderThin diet.

Drink Milk?

The human practice of consuming the milk (and products made therefrom) of other creatures has no parallel in nature. You will never see a baboon suckling at the teat of a wildebeest. And imagine trying to milk a wild buffalo by hand without the assistance of a high-powered tranquilizer gun. Only the technology of domestication makes it possible for us to drink the milk of another species.

Humans, like all mammals, consume the milk their mothers produce during lactation. Human milk, however, is quite different in composition from the milk of cud-chewing animals for sale on the grocer's shelf. The milk of herbivores (cows, goats, etc.) is designed for an entirely different sort of digestive system and often conflicts with that of humans. Many people are lactose-intolerant (see

Dahlqvist in Bibliography) or are intolerant to the acids produced as a by-product of milk digestion. Milk has also been shown to be among the top three food allergies (the other two are corn and wheat) found in tested individuals. The symptoms of milk allergy range from subtle (increased incidence of ear infection, loss of appetite, bad breath, irritability) to severe (abdominal cramping, eczema, colic, croup, diarrhea, constipation, asthma) and may be displayed even by lactose tolerant persons.

Although milk is often touted as an excellent source of calcium, milk drinkers worldwide have very high rates of osteoporosis and hip fractures, especially when compared to those (such as Japanese people eating their traditional diet) who obtain their calcium from other sources. This may be because excess consumption of calcium causes a deficiency of magnesium in the body, resulting in a reduction of bone density in later life (see Sojka and Evans in Bibliography). Another possible reason for reduced bone density is that most Americans don't eat enough leafy green vegetables rich in calcium. We also eat far fewer birds and fish than people with lower incidence rates of osteoporosis—all of which contain small bones that are hard to avoid when eating. Societal mores play a role in our not consuming bones. Unfortunately, in our culture it is generally considered uncouth to gnaw on bones in public.

Comparing the digestion of milk to the manufacture of common white glue can show another effect of milk on human digestion. Household glue is produced by exposing milk to acid and draining off excess fluid—a process very similar to human digestion. Indeed the hunter-gatherer will notice that consuming milk and dairy products results in a very gluey consistency in what comes out the other end. This stickiness may also result in constipation and flatulence.

Milk drinkers should not be concerned by the fat content of milk. The true culprits in milk are its sugars and foreign proteins. As low-fat dairy products contain less fat, which inhibits the absorption of sugars and foreign proteins, so with less fat both are absorbed more efficiently. Consequently, low-fat milk—a staple of obese Americans—actually has a much higher glycemic index (sugar content) than does whole milk and causes more severe reactions in lactose-intolerant persons.

In short, you don't need ruminant (cow, goat, etc.) milk to meet your calcium needs. You can derive plenty of calcium from regularly eating leafy green vegetables, nuts, and fish.

Sugar, It's Not So Sweet

Paleolithic humans rarely consumed refined sugar, except in the form of honey. The fruits they ate contained far less sugar than most of today's fruits, which have been bred for sweetness and larger size over hundreds of generations. The refined sugars that we gobble by the ton were unknown until very recently.

In adopting the NeanderThin diet, you must be careful not to replace sugar with other foods that are natural but contain almost as much sugar as refined products. Such foods include dried fruits and dried berries (especially raisins). You can eat them if the amount consumed does not exceed the amount of fresh fruit of the same kind that you would normally eat in a single serving. One small box of raisins would equal a rather substantial bunch of grapes. Similarly, two dried pear halves equal one whole pear.

Other Foods

The five categories of forbidden foods do not contain all of the fruits of technology. Others include certain gourds (e.g., squashes) and even a few nuts (e.g., cashews) that are inedible raw. When in doubt about any food, apply the basic principle of Paleolithic nutrition: Would this be edible when found in its natural state and without technology? If the food in question passes this test, it may be eaten without fear.

Don't Drink Alcohol

It is best not to consume alcohol in any amount from any source. Alcohol is a by-product of yeast digestion (the yeast equivalent of urine) and is known to damage the stomach, kidneys, and liver. Alcohol adds fat principally by producing cravings for both itself and other carbohydrates (see snack trays at any bar) and even other addictive substances (ask any former smoker). It is almost impossible to drink alcohol and follow the hunter-gatherer lifestyle. If you must drink, do so only on special occasions (once or twice a year) and stick to alcohols derived from fruit (wine and champagne). Be aware, however, that once you have been on the NeanderThin program for any length of time, drinking any form of alcohol could make you queasy. It is best to avoid alcohol altogether.

No Cheating Allowed

The NeanderThin program advises complete abstinence from the forbidden categories of food, because these foods have the inherent ability to produce cravings for themselves. Just as an alcoholic can't tolerate even a small quantity of drink, so the person who eats one potato chip may want many more—even several days later. After a week or so following the NeanderThin diet, cravings diminish considerably, only to return dramatically if cheating occurs.

Recent research into the pharmacology of food (see Wadley in Bibliography) presents a new perspective on food cravings. In the 1970s scientists began investigating the occurrence of druglike substances in grains and milk. Consuming these compounds provides a sense of well-being. Withdrawal symptoms appear when they are removed from the diet. People who exhibit the most physical intolerance to technology-dependent foods also exhibit the most severe withdrawal cravings. Ironically, those who have the most difficulties in adapting to the NeanderThin program have the most to gain from it.

As with any substance that produces cravings for itself, the degree of tolerance and the severity of withdrawal symptoms will vary among individuals. A few lucky people will find that occasionally cheating on the NeanderThin program causes no problem. Most, however, will find this to be a slippery slope leading to intense cravings, more cheating, and a sense of failure. Your personal tolerance for letting your dietary vigilance slip can only be determined through experimentation, following several weeks of avoiding the technology-dependent foods completely.

As you can see, we have eliminated much of what a typical person eats every day. Because an animal body cannot require that which in nature it cannot acquire, you won't be missing essential nutrients by following this diet plan. The forbidden fruits are found in most processed foods, so you will find yourself eating fewer and fewer of them. You will buy more raw foods in place of pre-packaged, manufactured foods. By eliminating processed, denatured foods from your diet, you will avoid forbidden fruits as well as the man-made preservatives, pesticides, and flavor-and-color enhancers relied upon by industrial food producers to maintain freshness and increase marketability.

CHAPTER SEVEN

Becoming a Modern Hunter-Gatherer

In spite of large geographic areas of the supermarket being off-limits to the modern hunter-gatherer, much of the food there is still fit for consumption. The foods found in a supermarket are unsurpassed in variety by those of any other culture since the Neolithic Revolution.

This variety is crucial to the hunter-gatherer lifestyle. By keeping our diet as varied as possible, we assure ourselves acquisition of all of the necessary nutrients, vitamins, minerals, and fiber we need for proper nutrition and energy production. By constantly seeking out new foods that fit within our criteria, we will stimulate our tastes and satisfy our need for new food experiences. We will also be following the example of our Paleolithic ancestors, who ate a much greater variety of foods than most modern people do.

Why a Meat-Based Diet Is Best

Meat is an important part of any healthy diet fed to a primate. Recent zoo studies have shown that monkeys fail to thrive or reproduce successfully when denied animal protein. For several thousand years man has, through technological progress in the chemical manipulation and combining of vegetable proteins, sought to eliminate the need for meat in the human diet. Despite these technological advances, modern vegetarians still often experience the developmental and reproductive difficulties displayed by meat-starved captive monkeys. In general, vegetarians exhibit the same high percentage of body fat as people eating an omnivorous agricultural diet. This wide range is not found within any species of wild animal or in hunter-gathering humans. Carnivorous peoples (e.g., Inuit Eskimo, African Samburu) and omnivorous peoples eating a hunter-gatherer diet (e.g., !Kung Bushmen and Australian aborigines) have a uniformly low percentage of body fat.

Persons undertaking vegetarian diet regimens often develop iron deficiency anemia, which causes lethargy and can lead to birth defects and mental retardation in children (see Scrimshaw in Bibliography). The vitamin and mineral deficiencies caused by a meatless diet have been well documented in the scientific literature (see Abrams in Bibliography). Without access to the forbidden foods and the supplements made possible by modern technology, it is impossible to meet the body's nutritional requirements eating a vegetarian diet. As evidence of this claim, consider that the human body cannot synthesize vitamin B_{12}, and, in nature, we can meet our B_{12} requirements only by eating meat.

There are no vegetarian primates in nature. In every film of primates in nature, you will see them eating meat. Nearly all primates get their animal protein from insects and other invertebrates, eggs, amphibians, reptiles, birds, and small mammals. Humans share these tastes, but because of our unique physical features we can also hunt and consume larger game. Our digestive systems have developed along with these features to enable us to utilize these food sources very efficiently. Many scientists think raw red meat provides the most complete source of nutrients for the human body (see Stefansson Studies section in Bibliography). It is the only single food capable of sustaining healthy human life when eaten exclusively, as is done by the Inuit (Eskimo), who eat little else during most of the year.

Many aboriginal North Americans and European explorers ate an exclusively raw meat diet in the form of pemmican. This high-energy food is produced by mixing extremely dried and powdered raw lean meat and hard animal fat in a one to one ratio. Eighty-five percent of the calories in pemmican are derived from fat, making it the closest nutritional equivalent to human mother's milk. Pemmican will keep for decades without refrigeration and can sustain a person without vitamin deficiency (scurvy, beriberi, etc.) indefinitely. It provides those who eat it with very high energy from very little consumption (½ to 1½ pounds per day if eaten exclusively). Because pemmican is almost entirely absorbed by the body (without the assistance of intestinal bacteria), very little waste results from its digestion (one sixth normal solid waste). The benefits of pemmican and other native foods so impressed the polar explorer Vilhjalmur Stefansson that he adopted the Inuit diet in his early twenties and kept to it nearly his entire life (he died at age eighty-three).

SHOULD I EAT RAW MEAT?

Although all meat is edible raw, you shouldn't eat supermarket meat raw. Proper care must be taken to cook or dry commercial meat to eliminate all bacterial contamination, which can cause food poisoning. Any of the vitamins destroyed by the cooking or drying process are easily replaced by eating fruits and vegetables.

Fat Is Good For You

The fat found in red meat is also an important component in the human diet. Without the high levels of glucose (blood sugar) produced by eating the forbidden fruits of technology, the body lacks energy for sustained exertion. Fat provides this source of energy by breaking down into glucose. Because this breakdown occurs only as needed, the body avoids the effects of high levels of blood sugar (diabetes), as well as extreme fluctuations in sugar levels (hypoglycemia).

Although some hunter-gatherers such as the Inuit eat considerably more fat than any Americans, they enjoy the lowest incidence of heart disease among all peoples. Many would attempt to explain this phenomenon as a genetically acquired trait, but this seeming immunity disappears when the Inuit abandon their traditional diet in favor of a civilized agricultural diet (which is much lower in dietary fat and cholesterol). It is easy to understand why when we realize that atherosclerotic disease is indicated by high blood glucose levels—not high cholesterol levels (see Abrams, De Bakey, and Reiser in Bibliography; see also pages 164–166).

The pancreas produces insulin in response to the presence of glucose in the blood. The liver, in turn, produces cholesterol in response to insulin in the blood. The body uses cholesterol to repair the damage done by excessive glucose to arterial walls and capillaries. Indeed, the highest rates of heart disease occur among those suffering from diabetes (excessively high glucose). Many of the other symptoms of diabetes are also caused by the damage done by glucose to the capillaries.

The NeanderThin convert may actually find that he or she is eating the same or less amounts of saturated fat than before. The absence of milk fat and hydrogenated vegetable oils will compensate for any increases in red meat consumption. Because the body must now draw on dietary and stored fat for energy, less fat will remain in the body for long periods of time. As time passes, the body will produce more of the enzymes needed to utilize fat resulting in more efficient use of both dietary fat and excess body fat. In this way weight loss, if necessary, is maximized.

Other sources of meat include poultry, fish, and small mammals, such as rabbits and squirrels. Invertebrates such as shellfish and crustaceans are also good sources of protein and minerals. They cannot, however, be used to eliminate all red meat as this will result in a substantial loss of energy due to lack of fat. In the absence of simple and complex carbohydrates, fat is vital as our main source of calories.

From Fruits to Nuts

Unlike the Inuit, most hunter-gatherers obtain a large portion of their food from plant foods, including the leaves, stems, and roots of plants that are edible raw, as well as from fruits, nuts, and berries.

Vegetables—i.e., edible leaves, stems, and roots—include lettuce, cabbage, spinach, celery, asparagus, onions, leeks, carrots, radishes, broccoli, cauliflower, edible mushrooms, and most herbs and spices (not an exhaustive list). All of these are edible uncooked and will provide the most nutrition when eaten raw by themselves or when combined into salads. They are only slightly less nutritious when cooked and can be used in soups, poultry stuffing, and as a hot side dish. Don't mistake grains, beans, and potatoes for Neander-friendly vegetables. Corn, green beans, and yams are not allowed.

Fruits include apples, peaches, pears, plums, apricots, avocados, bananas, melons, tomatoes, grapes, dates, figs, olives, citrus fruits, cherries, and many more varieties from all over the world. Most are now available year round thanks to modern transportation systems. All are edible raw and should be consumed when fresh, although dried fruits can be used as a convenient snack food if care is taken not to consume more than would be consumed in their fresh form. You should avoid canned fruits, candied fruits, preserves, jellies, and jams, as most contain very high amounts of sugar and have lost most of their nutrititive value during processing. If you are trying to lose body fat, you should limit your intake of fruits to levels available in the winter season, when the body is designed to burn fat.

Nuts are the edible seeds of trees and include walnuts, pecans, almonds, Brazil nuts, macadamias, acorns, chestnuts, hickory nuts, and many other varieties. Be careful, however, not to eat foods that are often mistakenly considered edible nuts. The peanut is a bean—not a nut. Peanuts are rich sources of aflatoxin, a highly carcinogenic substance. And the cashew, though a nut, is not edible raw. The cashew, a relative of the poison ivy plant, must be heated to neutralize the highly irritating oil in its shell before the nut can be extracted and eaten and thus is not allowed on NeanderThin. Though you can find many nuts in a roasted form, you should eat them raw whenever possible.

Although the following NeanderThin plan's Ten Commandments might seem restrictive, they aren't. There are a wealth of food choices available to the modern hunter-gatherer.

The Ten Commandments

DO EAT:	DON'T EAT:
Meats and Fish	Grains
Fruits	Beans
Vegetables	Potatoes
Nuts and Seeds	Dairy
Berries	Sugar

The Permitted Foods

What follows is a detailed list of the delicious foods available to you as you get started on the road to new eating habits and good health:

Meat and Fish

beef, veal, lamb, pork, venison, chicken, turkey, duck, pheasant, quail, rabbit, buffalo, moose, elk, seal, bear, squid, octopus, goose, oysters, clams, mussels, lobster, crayfish, halibut, cod, salmon, eel, trout, bass, carp, sardines, tuna, whitefish, orange roughie, all other fish, and any other form of meat or meat by-products such as lard (nonhydrogenated).

Fruits

apples, cherries, pears, peaches, melons, cucumbers, tomatoes, bananas, avocados, plums, olives, figs, dates, mangoes, kiwi, star fruit, pineapple, plums, pomegranates, passion fruit, peppers, watermelon, cantaloupe, honeydew melon, oranges, lemons, limes, tangerines, tangelos, citrons, nectarines, papaya, or any other fruit eaten fresh whenever possible.

Vegetables

lettuce, cabbage, kohlrabi, kale, rhubarb, cauliflower, flowers, broccoli, asparagus, parsley, spinach, celery, carrots, onions, mushrooms, greens, tea leaves, radish, leek, asparagus, endive, dandelion, brussels sprouts, artichoke, mint, basil, marjoram, oregano, rosemary, sage, thyme, fennel, onions, garlic, shallots, bay leaves, cloves, saffron, and any other part of a plant that is edible raw.

Nuts and Seeds

almonds, walnuts, pecans, Brazil, acorns, hickory, filberts, macadamia, flax, sesame, poppy, coriander, celery, anise, caraway, chervil, cumin, dill, fennel, mustard, and any others that are edible raw.

Berries

grapes, blueberries, raspberries, blackberries, boysenberries, strawberries, currants, and any others edible raw.

The Forbidden Foods

To get the most benefit from eating like our Paleolithic predecessors, there are foods you should avoid:

Grains

corn, wheat, barley, rye, rice, oats, millet, and all products made from them.

Beans

including all varieties of hard beans, lima beans, green beans, wax beans, peas, peanuts, chocolate, soy, fava beans, and all products made from them.

Potatoes

all varieties of potatoes and yams, beets, taro, cassava (tapioca), turnips, and all products made from them.

Dairy

milk, cheese, yogurt, whey, butter, and all products made from them—no matter what kind of animal milk was used to produce them.

Sugar

fructose, sucrose, maltose, dextrose, lactose, corn sweeteners, molasses, and all products made from them.

PART TWO

Living the NeanderThin Plan

CHAPTER EIGHT

Before Getting Started
on NeanderThin

Even though all of the natural foods outlined in the previous chapter are suitable for human nutrition, some considerations must be taken into account when seeking to emulate the diet of our Paleolithic ancestors.

These hunter-gatherers would have looked on a modern supermarket with wonder. Although seeing far fewer numbers of species of plants and animal than were available in their environment, Paleolithic humans would be confounded by the types of foods available in the same season. In the produce aisle, they would find summer fruits and vegetables. And in the meat section, they would find the flesh of fattened animals similar to the ones they hunted during the winter. Transportation advances of the twentieth century make this diversity of supermarket foods available. Using trucks, trains, ships, and planes, we gather our food from wherever it is in season and bring it to our tables.

Fruits, Veggies, Meat, and Fish

If you are seeking to lose weight or normalize your blood sugar, you should consider limiting your intake of summer fruits and vegetables in order to limit the effects of insulin resistance. These effects are made more severe when you are eating fruits and vegetables whose sugar content has been drastically increased through thousands of generations of selective breeding by farmers. Most wild fruits and vegetables have much more fiber and much less sugar than the domestic equivalents found in our supermarkets. To ensure that you get the most nutritional value from fruits and vegetables, choose those that are low in carbohydrates and high in fiber, such as green, cruciferous veggies. Reserve most sweet fruits for the occasional small-size desert or garnish. As different people display different levels of sensitivity to carbohydrates, some people may find that they need to maintain a "winter" diet (very low carbohydrate content) to maintain their desired percentage of body fat. But even people who are most sensitive to carbohydrates can occasionally indulge in sweet fruits or vegetables without experiencing bad long-term results.

The USDA's food pyramid recommends a daily intake of 5 servings of fruits and vegetables. However, many people find this amount of plant food to be more than they can conveniently eat during the day. It can also be difficult to eat 5 servings of fruits and vegetables every day while trying to follow a low-carbohydrate diet like NeanderThin. You can compromise by eating some fruits and vegetables (mostly green plants) and drinking several cups of green tea every day. A cup of green tea contains approximately one-quarter of the caffeine in a cup of coffee, meaning that a healthy person can drink 4 to 6 cups a day without experiencing negative effects. Green tea also happens to be loaded with phytochemicals and antioxidants (including vitamins C and E), making green tea a highly nutritious vegetable food. Among its many health benefits, regular consumption of green tea has been shown to protect against cardiovascular disease, several forms of cancer (e.g., digestive tract, skin, lung) and tooth decay. Black tea is higher in caffeine and is not as beneficial to health as is green tea (see Taylor in Bibliography).

When eating a very low-carb diet, a high percentage of dietary fat is necessary to maintain energy and health.* The Arctic explorer Vilhjalmur Stefansson found it easy to get at least 70 percent of his calories from fat when eating a diet composed only of domestic meat. The high fat intake required by a low-carb winter diet makes commercially raised meat seem ideal.

If our domestic meat were identical to the "fatted calf" of yore, a domestic, red-meat diet would be perfectly acceptable. Animals fattened on the grass of lush pastures or on silage feed (hay, alfalfa, etc.) have body fat compositions similar to their counterparts in the wild. Most animals fattened for American markets, however, are fed grain, due to profit considerations. Grain feeding fattens the animals very quickly during the last few weeks of their lives. But an all-grain diet is not normal for any grazing animal and leads to an abnormal ratio of omega-6 to omega-3 fatty acids in the composition of the animals' stored body fat.

It is virtually impossible for the average person to duplicate the diet of an Upper Paleolithic human. The animals that our Paleolithic ancestors hunted and ate are extinct. The nutritional profile of grain-fed meat is very different from that of wild-game meat. Wild-game meat exhibits a much healthier ratio of omega-6 to omega-3 fatty acids. The typical American eats a diet severely deficient in omega-3 fatty acids. Omega-3 deficiency has been linked to hormonal imbalances that can result in a host of health problems (elevated cholesterol, high blood pressure, chronic inflammatory diseases, diabetes, etc.). The average American's diet includes an omega-6/omega-3 ratio of 20 to 1 or greater. This ratio should be no greater than 4 to 1 (see Simopoulos in Bibliography). A ratio of between 2 to 1 and 1 to 1 is ideal.

Even though we can't rely on most commercially raised meat to get the right kinds and proportions of dietary fat, we have other

---

*The discussion of fatty acids and dietary fat in this chapter is based primarily on conversations with Dr. Loren Cordain of Colorado State University, a pioneer and leading authority in the field of Paleolithic nutrition.

alternatives. Fresh seafoods (primarily fatty fish like salmon, tuna, halibut, and herring), leafy green vegetables, walnuts, Brazil nuts, and flaxseeds all contain healthy doses of omega-3 fatty acids. Many egg producers are offering omega-3–enriched eggs, which are available at select health food markets and commercial grocery stores. Buffalo, longhorn, and emu meat—all of which have more healthy fatty acid profiles than standard commercial meats—are available as well.

If you prefer a more conveniently concentrated form of omega-3 fatty acids, you can purchase flaxseed and fish oil supplements in liquid and capsule forms. If you choose to go with fish oil, please be aware that cod liver oil (a staple of grandma's health regimen) contains potentially toxic quantities of vitamins A and D if the oil is taken in excessive doses. Look for fish oil supplements that contain EPA and DHA (daughter compounds of omega-3 fatty acids) without accompanying doses of vitamins A and D. The best fish oil supplements are derived from the flesh of salmon, herring, and mackerel.

Flaxseed oil is the richest plant source of omega-3 fatty acids (alpha-linolenic acid). Other plant-based omega-3 supplements, such as evening primrose and borage oils, contain significant quantities of omega-6 fatty acid. For this reason fish oil and flaxseed oil supplements are more desirable for the average person than evening primrose or borage oil supplements.

Omega-3 and omega-6 fatty acids fall into the category called polyunsaturated fatty acids (PUFA). The Paleolithic diet includes a healthy balance of saturated fatty acids (SFA's), monounsaturated fatty acids (MUFAs), and PUFAs (roughly a 1 to 2 to 1 ratio of these different kinds of fats). Within NeanderThin guidelines, the richest sources of SFAs are red meat and eggs. Coconut oil and palm oil are also high in SFAs. The most common dietary sources of MUFA's include olives (fruit and oil), avocados (fruit and oil), almonds, macadamia nuts, and hazelnuts.

Your primary sources of fat should be olive oil, avocados, lean meats, seafood (especially fatty fish), MUFA-rich nuts (see previous paragraph), walnuts, Brazil nuts, omega-3–enriched eggs, and flaxseed oil. If the majority of your fat calories come from these foods, you will ensure that your dietary ratio of omega-6 to omega-3 fatty acids and your overall dietary fat ratio (SFA/MUFA/PUFA) will be nutritionally balanced. These foods should account for at least 35 percent of your total daily intake of calories.

Many health-conscious people are especially concerned about eating too much saturated fat (SFAs). If your diet is composed mostly of foods rich in omega-3 fatty acids and MUFAs, your SFA intake will be regulated as a side effect. If you choose to regularly eat commercially produced grain-fed beef, chicken, and pork, try to limit yourself to the leanest cuts of these meats. Don't eat the skin on your chicken or turkey. Trim visible fat as much as possible. Buy low-fat ground beef. Ideally, your meat selections would consist of fresh fish, wild game, and range-fed animals such as bison (buffalo), emu, and longhorn cattle. You will probably find that by eating more monounsaturated and omega-3 fats, your taste will naturally shift to leaner cuts of meat.

Meat Allergies

Another issue that relates to eating grain-fed meat is the phenomenon of meat allergy. For example, many Americans display allergies to beef. Since humans evolved to eat the meat and fat of grass eaters, an allergy to beef would seem to make no sense. This seeming contradiction may be explained by the fact that when a cow eats corn, some of the corn proteins become transferred to the cow's meat. So when a person with grain intolerance (celiac disease) eats grain-fed beef and experiences an allergic reaction, he may be reacting to the corn protein in the meat instead of the meat itself.

Another example: A group of people eating soy-fed beef experienced anaphylactic shock symptoms (allergic reaction). The problem was the source of the soy fed to the cattle. In an attempt to protect soybeans from blight, the soybeans were genetically spliced with a Brazil nut gene that was supposed to confer upon the soybeans greater immunity to the blight. The people who had allergic reactions to the experimental animals' meat were severely allergic to Brazil nuts. For this reason all strains of this soybean were withdrawn from testing. In short, people with allergies to the foods that are fed to commercially raised cattle may want to seek alternate sources of meat.

Becoming NeanderThin

In a sense, it is contradictory to discuss a NeanderThin "plan." In nature, humans follow only the dictates of their environment in meeting their needs for water, food, clothing, and shelter. In the course of securing these necessities, hunter-gatherers ate only the foods they were designed by nature to eat. And their daily routine included moderate amounts of physically strenuous activities that eliminated their need for additional exercise. Hunter-gatherers didn't follow a rigid pattern of diet or exercise. They just did what nature required for their survival, and the result was good health. If they didn't succumb to death as the result of trauma, infectious disease, or the perils of childbirth, hunter-gatherers could expect to live as long as modern affluent humans without suffering from the degenerative conditions that plague our elderly populations.

We modern humans, however, have come to rely on technology for everything we do. We have banking, legal, medical, transportation, and other systems for the simplest activities. We are systems freaks. Without a system, any large task seems unmanageable to us. So the NeanderThin plan detailed in this chapter is provided as a quick-start guide. It's not a rigid plan, but a set of loose guidelines to get you on the path to a more natural way of eating and living. Once you have been following NeanderThin for a few weeks, you will begin to customize the Paleolithic diet/lifestyle to meet your individual needs.

The following steps to becoming NeanderThin are listed in order of importance. If you don't want to make the transition immediately, you can gradually implement the steps in the order listed.

1. Make a commitment. At first, NeanderThin may seem to be a difficult program to practice, but in reality it's very easy. Even the most undisciplined people (the author, for example) can follow this plan if they can get through the first week without cheating. This book will tell you everything you need to know to ensure your success. And by following up with your own research you will be further convinced of the validity of the NeanderThin program. Whether you are slim and in good health or ill and overweight, the benefits you will experience in just a few weeks will give you the resolve to stick with the program.

To begin with, simply resolve that for some period of time you will not eat any grains, beans, potatoes, milk, or refined sugar. A three-week commitment would be ideal, but most people find a one-week commitment to be easily achievable. People with experience in 12-step programs may want to take it one day at a time. However long you commit to stay on the diet, stick with it religiously. Otherwise, your results will be unpredictable. You must give your body a reasonably extended period of time to acclimate to the NeanderThin diet.

2. Give up the forbidden fruits. Clear out any grains, beans, dairy, potatoes, and sugar (and products made from them) in your refrigerator, freezer, and pantry. Donate packaged goods to a local food bank if you wish. By removing all technology-dependent foods from your kitchen, you simplify the task of breaking old habits by removing any possible source of temptation. (Don't forget condiments!)

The basic components of the NeanderThin diet—meats, vegetables, nuts, fruits, and berries—are listed and explained in earlier chapters. Refer to the Ten Commandments (page 58) for a list of foods to eat and foods to avoid. As long as you stay within the list of acceptable foods, you can eat as much and as often as you want. Hunger is a sign that your body is storing fat. Don't go hungry. The more NeanderThin-friendly foods you eat, the faster your metabolism will be. The faster your metabolism, the more energy you will have and the easier it will be for you to lose weight (if you need to). See the menu suggestions (page 150) and the recipe section (page 111) for satisfying snack and meals plans.

3. Limit carbohydrate intake. Fruits and carbohydrate-rich vegetables are certainly acceptable in the NeanderThin program, but people who find themselves unable to maintain fat loss are usually eating too many of these sugary foods. If your goal is to lose weight, it is best to choose fruits and vegetables that have a fairly low sugar content. Choose pears, oranges, plums, and berries over bananas, mangoes, and dates. Choose leafy greens, celery, broccoli, and cauliflower over carrots. Favor fresh-squeezed juices (preferably with pulp) over highly processed, concentrated juices (which are really just fruit sugar water). Eating any food raw will minimize the amount of sugar your body will absorb from the food. Choose raw fruits and vegetables over steamed, cooked, or canned varieties. To maximize safe fat loss in a small amount of time, remove fruit and sugary vegetables from your diet or at least limit your intake of sugary plant foods to minuscule amounts (e.g., half a pear a day) until you reach your desired body composition. In doing so you will be modeling your diet after that of hunter-gatherers to whom fruit is available only seasonally.

Giving up sweets may be one of the hardest things for many people who would attempt to abide by the guidelines of the

NeanderThin diet. However, once you have reached your desired percentage of body fat, you can begin to add carbohydrate-rich foods to your diet in small amounts. To make up for the loss of chocolate cake and cheesecake, try frozen fruit juice or fruit salads. Frozen berries also make a delicious dessert. A fruit smoothie made in a blender with ice, bananas, and other fresh fruits is a good substitute for a milkshake. And frozen bananas taste similar to ice cream. Honey, if used at all, should be used sparingly—no more than a few teaspoons a week. In time, your sensitivity to natural sugar will increase to the point that raw fruit and small amounts of honey will totally satisfy any desire for sweets that you may have. Not only will any cravings you might have for chocolate and candy disappear, should you try to eat these foods you will probably find that the extraordinary amounts of refined sugar they contain are too much for the newly developed sensitivity of your taste buds.

In short, don't eat lots of carbohydrate-rich fruits and vegetables every day. Most of your calories should come from meats, nuts, seeds, and oils. Rely on green vegetables, raw nuts and seeds, and small amounts of low-sugar fruits for the plant-based part of your diet.

4. Increase fat consumption. A common mistake made by neophyte hunter-gatherers is trying to limit their fat intake. Limiting dietary fat on a low-carbohydrate diet such as NeanderThin will only result in extreme hunger and fatigue and will actually slow any needed weight loss by lowering your metabolism. If you have a high-energy day planned, have more meat or eggs at breakfast. Snack throughout the day on high-fat foods such as sardines, canned salmon (low salt), nuts, seeds, or pemmican to boost your energy.

As your body adapts to the NeanderThin routine, fat will become more attractive to your taste. Feel free to indulge this new taste whenever possible (being careful, of course, to avoid fats that are not on the diet—i.e., oils and fats derived from beans, grains, and milk). If you have eaten a meatless and/or low-fat diet for any length of time, it may take your system a week or so to begin producing the necessary amount of digestive enzymes to handle your new diet. Since we are designed by nature to eat a high-fat diet, you will find that your taste for fat need not be acquired. All that is necessary is that you refine your taste for fat to include the different kinds of fats eaten by our Paleolithic ancestors. After your body acclimates to your new diet, only psychological barriers would keep you from enjoying foods high in fat.

The Arctic explorer Stefansson learned firsthand of the effects of fat deprivation combined with a low-carbohydrate diet. He detailed a condition resulting from such a diet, saying,

> If you are transferred suddenly from a diet normal in fat to one consisting wholly of . . . [lean meat] you eat bigger and bigger meals for the first few days until at the end of about a week you are eating in pounds three or four times as much as you were at the beginning of the week. By that time you are showing signs both of starvation and protein poisoning. You eat numerous meals; you feel hungry at the end of each; you are in discomfort through distension of the stomach with much food; and you begin to feel a vague restlessness. Diarrhoea will start in from a week to 10 days and will not be relieved unless you secure fat. Death will result after several weeks. (See Speth in Bibliography.)

5. Drink lots of fresh water. The human body is approximately 70 percent water. It cannot be stressed enough that you should try to consume as much pure water as is possible. Water is essential for the elimination of waste and other body processes. Concerns about bowel functioning arise frequently among people making the transition to NeanderThin. At first you may notice a change in the frequency and/or consistency of your bowel movements. Drinking lots of water will help to normalize your elimination cycle. After a few weeks on the diet, your bowel movements should be regular. In this regard, it is important that you always have ready access to a source of purified water. If you are thirsty and only chlorinated water is available, then drink it. It is better to drink than to go thirsty, but stick to purified water as much as possible. Use purified water for teas or any cooking that may require water—not only is purified water healthier, but it will improve taste as well. When eating, however, try to limit the amount of liquids you drink, so as to avoid disrupting the digestion of your food. Also remember that juices and teas aren't substitutes for pure water. The tired admonition of drinking at least 8 glasses of water a day still stands. Two to four liters or more per day is highly recommended.

6. Increase physical activity. One of the chief pitfalls of modern life is the tendency toward being sedentary. The effect of such a lifestyle is a degeneration of the body's ability to meet physical demands placed upon it. After a period of time (determined by your physical condition upon adopting the hunter-gatherer diet), your body will adjust to its natural weight, body composition, and metabolism. To keep your muscles and bones strong, you need to engage in regular physical activity. This doesn't mean that you necessarily have to adopt a rigorous exercise program (unless you so desire). All that is necessary is regular exercise of some kind. This may mean simply adding more activity to daily events: parking farther from the store than usual or taking the stairs instead of the elevator. The primary activity of hunting and gathering is walking and observing—learn to do both. True hunter-gatherers are light on their feet and aware of their environment. In this respect, the best physical activities are the ones that allow you to develop a stronger awareness of and relationship with your world. Activities such as picking berries, birdwatching, hunting, and foraging for mushrooms or wild herbs require that you be "tuned in" to your environment. You can't just don a set of headphones and forget about the rest of the world. Although health clubs and gyms certainly are avenues to fitness, the best exercise is the kind for which you don't have to change your clothes. If you are interested in pursuing an organized program of exercise (highly recommended for optimum results), see Chapter 10, Becoming NeanderFit: A Five-Week Program (page 87).

The NeanderThin plan is relatively simple to follow. You eat as much as you want of the acceptable natural foods. You don't have to count calories. You don't have to worry about portion sizes. You need to exercise only moderately. And you can customize the entire program to fit the demands of your lifestyle. After a few weeks of following the program religiously, it will become second nature to you. You will learn how to accommodate your dietary needs in any situation. You will naturally want to be more physically active to release the excess energy you will have. And the results you will achieve in a relatively short amount of time will provide you with the necessary motivation to make the NeanderThin plan a lifestyle change as opposed to a short-term crash diet. The next chapter includes several tips on how to make NeanderThin a permanent part of your life.

CHAPTER NINE

Mosaic of Diet Tips

Many seeming challenges face a hunter-gatherer living in the midst of an agricultural society. But as we have seen, modern transportation makes possible a diet with great variety, so you should not feel that you will be limited in your choice of foods within the guidelines of the NeanderThin diet. Even though you might be giving up a number of your favorite foods, keep in mind the benefits of eating only food you are designed to eat, as well as the fact that on this diet you can eat as much as you want of those foods. Just think! All you can eat—and you don't have to watch your waistline!

Being a modern hunter-gatherer is really quite simple in this land of grocery stores and cafeterias. But it does require that you rethink your approach to everyday eating. You can no longer wolf down burgers and fries on the way to a meeting. Take-out Chinese is no longer an option. So here are some tips concerning how to go about your hunting and gathering in a successful fashion:

Understand why you are giving up the "forbidden fruits"
You don't have to be a medical doctor or a scientist to understand the scientific reasoning behind the Paleolithic diet. The scientific arguments for adopting this diet are provided in layperson's

terms in the earlier chapters of this book. Make sure you understand them. Go to your local library, and do your own research using the Bibliography at the end of the book. Not only will you then be better able to explain why you don't want the baked potato that comes with your steak, you will understand why the diet works, as well as how you stand to benefit from it. This understanding will make it much easier to stick with NeanderThin.

"You mean you don't eat bread?"

To most people the idea that bread, corn, cheese, and potatoes should not be eaten is unfathomable. Almost everything that is said today about nutrition would lead us to believe that our diets should consist of lots of complex carbohydrates and little fat. So telling people that you do not eat grains, beans, potatoes, sugar, and dairy products is likely to make you appear a bit strange. Be aware that to see why technology-dependent foods are not fit for human consumption requires a paradigm shift in your viewpoint on nature, nutrition, and health. The NeanderThin program turns upside down the common wisdom concerning what humans should eat to be fit, trim, and healthy. As was previously stated, it is helpful to gain a basic understanding of the scientific evidence that supports the hunter-gatherer diet. Your understanding will help you to explain to people concisely in layperson's terms why a diet seemingly high in animal fat will not clog your arteries or give you cancer. If you wish to avoid such discussions, just tell people that you are unable to digest these foods and that they make you sick. Chances are that you will not be lying if you have been following the NeanderThin program for any length of time.

Many NeanderThin converts have found that their enthusiasm for their new lifestyle borders on fanaticism. If you find yourself unable to resist the urge to proselytize, don't think you're alone. Paleolithic nutrition needs all the press and word-of-mouth support it can get. Your advocacy of the NeanderThin plan will help to raise people's awareness that the conventional dietary wisdom (low-fat, high-carbohydrate) is outdated. The act of defending your way of life will also strengthen your resolve and commitment to stay NeanderThin. But don't be too overbearing. The idea is not to win arguments at the expense of alienating misinformed people. Instead, try to win their allegiance by providing valuable, accurate information based on sound scientific research. Of course, it's always better to lead by example than to just preach at people. Your results from eating NeanderThin should be your best argument.

Share the hunter-gatherer lifestyle with your spouse or a friend

Upon making the decision to adopt the hunter-gatherer way of eating and living, you may find it difficult not to give in to temptations when they arise. When everyone else at the party is drinking or having cake, you may feel isolated—as if you are missing out. By sharing your new way of eating and looking at the world with those who are close to you, you can create a base of support that will make it easier for you to stick to the diet. You will also be helping others to see the benefits of being a modern hunter-gatherer, possibly convincing those whom you care about to adopt a healthier diet. Seeing the success of your friends and family members on the plan will also strengthen your commitment to the program.

Variety

By constantly changing the foods you eat every day, you will find your new diet to be more interesting and easier to follow. Also, by varying your diet you will realize a greater intake of necessary vitamins and minerals.

Wild game

Having lived in their natural habitats, wild animals are better sources of meat for humans than are domesticated animals, which are raised typically on grains and sometimes given injections of steroids and antibiotics. Meat from wild game is likely to be purer than meat from domesticated animals. All animals thrive on a natural diet. The animal that lives its entire life on a natural diet will have a healthier body with a more beneficial lean-to-fat tissue composition, amino acids, and enzymes. The balance of essential fatty acids in game meat is healthier than in commercial meat. Wild game usually tastes better as well.

The act of hunting or fishing will also give you a more direct, spiritual connection to your food. By becoming an active part of the food chain, you will be more aware of your role in nature and have a greater interest in preserving wild places.

Wild plants

Hunting and gathering your own food provides a closer, more intimate relationship with your world. By foraging for berries, wild mushrooms, herbs, roots, and other wild plants, you develop a closer connection to the natural world. You will see how the plants that are an important part of your diet have an even more important role as parts of a complex ecological system, and that, as a human being, you too have an environmental niche—that you are an integral, inseparable part of the natural world. (Note: Don't eat wild plants harvested within 50 feet of roads or other urban developments. Such plants may be contaminated with toxic pollutants.)

Balanced fat intake

As was stated in the previous chapter, you should not be afraid of eating fat. NeanderThin is a moderate- to high-fat diet, as is the diet of any human living in nature. But in nature the kinds of fats we eat are naturally balanced. That is, a natural diet includes a healthy balance of the essential (polyunsatured) fatty acids (EFAs) and of the three categories of fat (saturated, monounsaturated, and polyunsatured). Commercial meat tends to be deficient in omega-3 fatty acids, so if you eat commercially raised meat, you must supplement your diet with foods rich in healthy fats. To that end you will want to include large amounts of nuts (walnuts, Brazil nuts, hazelnuts, macadamias, etc., not peanuts or cashews), avocados, olive oil, and fatty fish in your diet. You can also supplement your diet with flaxseed and fish oils to meet your EFA requirements. An EFA deficiency can lead to significant problems, so maintaining a healthy balance in your dietary fat is very important. Avoid cod liver oil, as it can easily become spoiled and usually contains high levels of vitamins A and D (these vitamins can have a toxic effect on the body in excessive quantities).

Eating out

At first it might seem that most restaurants are off limits to the urban hunter-gatherer. To be sure, you will find yourself at a loss when trying to order from the menu at your typical hamburger-and-fries joint. Most fast food restaurants will be useless to you. Many use hydrogenated vegetable oil—a substance that you should definitely avoid—in cooking their meals. Italian and Asian restaurants may also prove difficult. Cafeterias, organic restaurants, steak and barbecue houses, and seafood restaurants are all good bets. Most Mexican restaurants serve fajitas, which can be eaten without the tortillas, beans, and rice that are usually served with a fajita dinner. And most dining establishments will have a selection of salads from which to choose. If you will be eating out with friends at a restaurant that will make it difficult to remain on the diet, eat something before you go and order a salad—without the dressing, cheese, and croutons of course. Also, don't hesitate to customize an order or ask for substitutions. After all, you are the customer and the restaurant staff is there to serve you. As a hunter-gatherer, eating out may cost more than usual, but the money that you will save on doctor bills, medicine, and a new wardrobe every six months (to accommodate your increasing girth) will more than compensate.

On the road

Traveling should provide no inescapable problems for the foresighted and resourceful hunter-gatherer. If you know that you will be going to a place where it will be difficult to find hunter-gatherer fare, then plan on taking some trail mix (nuts and dried fruit), beef jerky, pemmican (refer to the Pemmican section) or any other such convenient foods. No matter where you are, you can almost always find a restaurant that serves bacon and eggs, or salad and steak. Remember to carry a bottle of water. And don't forget to eat lots of foods (fish, avocados, nuts, seeds, green vegetables, etc.) that contain substantial amounts of monounsaturated fat and essential fatty acids. While on the road you may want to take supplements of flaxseed or fish oil to ensure that you meet your EFA requirements.

Pemmican

The hunter-gatherer's miracle food, pemmican, makes practicing the NeanderThin program easy. If eaten exclusively, a small amount per day (¾ pound for the average adult) will sustain you indefinitely without vitamin or mineral deficiencies. It provides quick energy without filling your stomach. It's easy to digest (95 percent absorbed in digestion) and produces almost no waste. Since the digestion of pemmican requires no intestinal flora, eating pemmican exclusively for several days will greatly reduce bacterial presence in the gut. Pemmican is almost totally absorbed by the body. Very little waste remains from its digestion. As such, pemmican is an excellent first solid food for infants, and a good choice for anyone suffering from a gastrointestinal disorder.

Invented by aboriginal North Americans and used for centuries by French-Canadian fur traders, pemmican consists of equal parts raw, dehydrated, powdered red meat and tallow (rendered animal fat). Building on these basic ingredients, you can customize pemmican to your taste, including spices, nuts, dried berries, etc.

Pemmican is easy to carry (it's highly concentrated), requires no refrigeration or preservatives, and provides quick energy. It's the perfect food when you don't have enough time to eat a full meal. It's also the perfect workout food for the NeanderThin athlete who can't carbo-load. The taste of pemmican may be unfamiliar at first, but most people who try it eventually find themselves craving it.

Snacking

The NeanderThin rule concerning snacking is very simple: If you are hungry, eat. Eat as much as it takes to satisfy your hunger. With this rule in mind, keep plenty of low-sugar fruits (e.g., pears, oranges, melons) and sliced veggies around. A big bowl of trail mix (with small amounts of dried fruit, if any) is definitely invaluable. Cold roast beef, a handful of nuts, or a can of sardines (packed in water, olive oil, or tomato sauce). Just be sure that your snack foods are within the dietary guidelines—could I eat this if I were naked with a sharp stick on the savanna? An occasional bag of potato chips or cookies may seem harmless, but nothing will serve better to sabotage your efforts than partaking of small amounts of these forbidden fruits. Also, make sure that you aren't eating a lot of sugar in the form of fruit when snacking, as this can pack on the pounds.

Read labels

In the course of changing to a diet not based on technology-dependent foods, you will find yourself relying less and less on packaged foods. In the event that you continue to buy boxed or canned foods, read labels to make sure that the foods contain no grain by-products (e.g., rice syrup, high fructose corn syrup, cornstarch, etc.), bean by-products (e.g., soy, soy protein, soy sauce, peanut oil, etc.), or added sugars (e.g., sucrose, fructose, maltose, dextrose, lactose, artificial sweeteners, etc.). Remember also that the ingredients will be listed in order from greatest to least amount present in the product. In other words, a product with soy as the fifth ingredient is less troublesome than a product with soy as the first or second ingredient. Of course, you will also want to avoid any food that is treated with chemical preservatives, additives, or food coloring agents. Hydrogenated vegetable oil, an ingredient used to improve the consistency and taste of many processed foods, is a carcinogenic substance that you should avoid, more so even than synthetic chemicals. Shopping at health food stores and natural food stores will simplify your search for pure foods and make it much easier to find high-quality sources of the meats and produce that will constitute the majority of your diet.

Artificial sweeteners

When any very sweet substance is consumed, the digestive and metabolic systems must be prepared before it reaches the stomach. The trigger mechanism for these changes is in the tongue. The taste of sweetness will slow the metabolic rate, alter the delicate balance of digestive enzymes, and produce cravings—whether the sweetness comes from an artificial or a "natural" sweetener. Many artificial sweeteners have also been found to be carcinogenic, and you should avoid them for that reason alone.

Alcohol

Many people are thrown off the NeanderThin program by their inability to abstain from alcohol. Nachos and pizza seem almost inseparable from beer (the craving for each is caused by the same chemical reaction in the brain). And who drinks wine at cocktail parties without eating cheese? People who claim to be only social drinkers should remember that drinking tea or orange juice, while everyone else has wine or beer or something stronger, allows them to get more of what they socially drink for in the first place. Being alert while others are slightly inebriated or drunk leaves you in a better position to get a date or impress a potential client in the midst of your competitors.

Salt

As a hunter-gatherer, your taste for salt should diminish. Over-consumption of salt causes the body to retain water, thereby increasing blood pressure. On the NeanderThin diet you will get enough sodium by eating meat.

Processed meats

Processed meats such as hot dogs, bacon, sausage, and lunch meats are not exclusively forbidden. You should, however, avoid supermarket varieties, which are prepared with sugar, corn syrup, salt, and chemical preservatives. Besides being unhealthy, these preservative technologies have become obsolete in the presence of modern refrigeration. If you cannot find a first-class butcher capable of making untainted varieties of these meats, make your own (which also happens to be far less expensive). Don't make processed meats a daily staple. Have them occasionally as a treat if you wish. Most of the meat you eat should be unprocessed.

Eggs

Wild birds' eggs are the most preferable, free-range birds' eggs are the next most favorable, and factory-farm eggs are the least desirable. This is because the balance of amino acids and essential fatty acids is more favorable in the wild and free-range eggs. For this reason, people who have experienced egg allergies may find wild and free-range eggs to be more compatible with their digestion. People have debated whether fertile or infertile eggs are better. And while it is true that fertile eggs are actually healthier, the reason has nothing to do with the fertilization process. The difference is in what is fed to the mother. Eggs that are bred for fertility require a completely different and nutritionally superior food mixture in comparison to eggs that are bred for food production. Eggs fortified with omega-3 fatty acids are also closer to wild eggs in nutrition.

Coffee

In reality a burnt berry, coffee is popularly referred to as a bean. Because it is not edible raw, it is forbidden on the NeanderThin program. To avoid the pangs of caffeine withdrawal, substitute tea for coffee. The darker teas are higher in caffeine than green teas, but green teas are preferable, as they are not fermented. Use caution with herbal teas as some have side effects. Some work as laxatives, diuretics, sedatives, and stimulants (e.g., ephedrine in Ma Huang tea). Some teas can even be toxic if consumed daily over a long period of time (e.g., goldenseal). Try teas derived from mint or rose hips.

Detoxify your living environment

Although the focus of this book is cleansing your inner environment of foreign proteins introduced through improper diet, there are many things you can do to improve the conditions of your immediate external environment. Man is not designed to live in a sealed box for seventy years, so keep your house clean and filled with fresh air. Install a HEPA air filtration system if you can afford one. Also, try to use fewer industrial cleaners in your home, switching to natural or "organic" cleansing agents available at most health food stores. Buy a water purification system for your home, and avoid contact with soaps and other hygienic products made with synthetic chemicals. There are many books available on detoxifying your home. Educate yourself and take action to make your living and working environments as toxin-free as possible.

Hormonal imbalances

Women on birth control drugs or hormone replacement therapy during menopause may have problems losing body fat, as these therapies mimic pregnancy and cause the body to retain fat. This effect may be overcome by lowering the dosage of estrogen, adding small doses of the hormone testosterone, or by the elimination of synthetic hormones altogether (the most natural solution). See your doctor before undertaking any changes to the dosage of your prescribed medication.

Men taking female hormones or who have had one or both testicles removed for treatment of prostate or testicular cancer cannot pursue these options. The drawbacks of these therapies, however, can also be overcome by regular, strenuous exercise.

Sunlight

The common admonitions of the medical community to avoid sunlight exposure should be taken with a grain of salt. Sunlight provides the basis for organic life on earth. The photosynthetic process in plants is totally dependent upon sunlight, and plants constitute the collective lungs of humanity. As such, we are dependent upon the sun for our every breath. Exposure to sunlight enables the body to synthesize vitamin D, which is essential to human life. As was discussed earlier, man is designed to be active during daylight hours. Provided by nature with an onboard air-conditioning system (the ability to sweat profusely), he can keep from overheating even while engaged in strenuous activities during the hottest hours of the day. So do not be afraid to go out in the sun. Overexposure (e.g., sunbathing) should be avoided of course, but, depending upon your skin type, a moderate amount of daily exposure to the sun is completely natural and should be welcomed—not avoided.

If your job requires you to spend most of your time indoors, you might consider the following ruse to get some time outdoors. Buy a pack of cigarettes, and tell your boss you've recently started smoking. Start taking five-minute breaks every hour during which you go outside to get some sun and fresh air. Of course, you shouldn't actually smoke.

And finally . . .

Don't cheat!

Upon making the transition from a diet high in complex carbo-hydrates to one based on large amounts of animal protein and ani-mal fat, "treating" yourself to a bag of potato chips, a bowl of ice cream, or your favorite Mexican dish will have the opposite effect that it once did. What was once a satisfying meal or snack will prob-ably make you sick. Carbohydrates have an addictive effect, and once you have given them up, indulging yourself may send you reeling. Because the immune system responds to even small doses, the smallest amounts of forbidden fruit may produce weight gains far out of proportion to their size. Some NeanderThin neophytes have reported gaining several pounds after eating only a single serv-ing of rice or a small piece of cake. Some people will find that they can tolerate an occasional lapse in dietary discipline. But if you are like most people, you will find that if you can't stick to the diet reli-giously, you are better off not adopting it at all.

If and when you do cheat (face it—we all cheat sooner or later), don't feel that all is lost and that you can't continue the NeanderThin program. Depending on the amount and kind of forbidden fruit(s) consumed, there will probably be a period of time where you will feel uncomfortable, if not ill. Your discomfort or illness should not last very long. Continue to pursue the NeanderThin program, and before long, you will be back on track. An infrequent lapse in dietary vigilance can serve as excellent reinforcement for the devoted hunter-gatherer's commitment to his or her body and envi-ronment. This is not to say that any amount of cheating is encour-aged or is advisable. Just remember that we are all human.

CHAPTER TEN

Becoming NeanderFit: A Five-Week Program

The first copy of *NeanderThin* (a photocopied manuscript) was sold to a body builder. Over the years the authors have consulted with many athletes. We have also benefited from the work of Dr. Arthur De Vany (professor of economics at UC-Irvine, author of *Evolutionary Fitness*) and Dr. Del Thiessen (professor of evolutionary psychology at the University of Texas, author of *Survival of the Fittest*). Our approach to exercise is based on studies of the physical activity patterns of hunter-gatherers. And while it may seem contradictory for two 6-feet tall, 145-pound computer nerds to discuss fitness and exercise, let us assure you that both of us are fit and exhibit good muscle definition. Our combined percentage of body fat is less than 12 percent.

In nature, hunter-gatherers don't spend a lot of time doing strenuous physical labor. At most, they work 2 to 3 hours per day (even in the harshest environments) to meet their food, clothing, and shelter needs. Unlike the 10- to 12-hour, physically exhausting regimen of the Neolithic farmer, Paleolithic hunter-gatherers didn't do the same thing every day. Different levels of physical stress were called for at different times of the year. Spring and summer are naturally more active times of the year than fall and winter.

Hunter-gatherers eat the most fat and calories and are the leanest, best-toned population groups in the world. In the course of his or her daily routine, a hunter-gatherer usually burns fewer calories than does a person playing a leisurely round of golf (carrying his or her own clubs). So it's not necessary to train like a professional athlete to reach a high level of fitness. To keep your body toned and fit, you can simply add more physical activity to your daily routine. To maximize weight loss and greatly enhance your physical fitness, it is best to engage in a loosely organized program of moderate exercise similar to the activity patterns of our prehistoric ancestors.

The physical demands of Stone Age life occurred chaotically. The rigors of the hunt did not follow any schedule. Instead, hunter-gatherers went through short periods in which hard intensive labor was required, interspersed within longer periods of moderate activity and no activity at all. In tailoring an exercise program for yourself, try to break your workouts up into several intense sessions at random intervals per month, three or fewer per week, supplemented by several moderate workouts. Also include days during which you "play," and others during which you don't have much physical activity at all.

By intense exercise we mean, primarily, weight training. Bodybuilders and professional wrestlers have, since the sixties, used high-fat, high-protein diets to achieve maximum muscle gain with a minimum increase in body fat. If you want to build muscles, NeanderThin combined with a weight training regimen will greatly accelerate the process. The resulting increase in muscle bulk will increase your metabolic rate whether or not you engage in regular aerobic exercise. Besides following the NeanderThin diet, building muscle is the best thing you can do to lose body fat.

Paleo-Aerobics

The reason to exercise aerobically is not for weight loss but to improve your cardiovascular stamina. Aerobic exercise doesn't have to be intense to be effective. Recent research by Dr. Kenneth Cooper at the Cooper Clinic in Dallas, Texas, even indicates that regular periods of intense aerobic exercise may be dangerous. Moderate amounts of aerobic exercise, including walking, jogging, swimming, low-impact aerobics, and bicycling, are much safer. The best exercise for you will be the kind you enjoy the most. Hunter-gatherers play a lot because they have a lot of free time on their hands. Sports like basketball, kick-boxing, judo, golf, softball, and volleyball combine short periods of intense activity with longer periods of moderate or no activity. The physical effects of these kinds of activities are similar to the kind of physical exertion experienced while hunting and gathering. Be sure to play a lot.

NeanderFit: The Plan

The following exercise diary is an example of a "chaotic" exercise program. The plan covers a five-week period. You can use it as a guide to creating your own exercise program, or you can follow the outlined program exactly as written. Whatever you do, make sure that you don't overdo it. If you haven't been exercising regularly for a while, you might want to visit your doctor and have a physical examination before beginning any new exercise program.

WEEK 1
Monday

warm-up: 5 minutes walking (walk on treadmill or outdoors)
5 to 10 minutes stretching (focus on upper body)
30 minutes weight lifting
At the beginning of the program, you will want to take it easy. Do 1 exercise for each upper body part. For each exercise do 1 set of 12 to 15 repetitions using light weight. Don't rest more than 1 minute between each exercise.

- bench presses
- triceps extensions
- bicep curls
- shoulder presses
- seated row
- abdominal crunches (modified sit-ups with legs bent and feet in the air or supported on a chair or bench)
- back extensions (begin by lying on your stomach; raise your upper body from the floor until you can look at the ceiling; lower yourself to the ground; repeat)

5 to 10 minutes stretching (cooldown)

You should be able to finish the warm-up, weight lifting, and cooldown in about 45 minutes.

Tuesday

warm-up: 5 minutes light stretching

20 to 30 minutes walking at moderate pace

5 to 10 minutes stretching

It is always preferable to exercise outdoors if you live in a reasonably smog-free area. Use a treadmill if the weather precludes you from walking outside. If you have been moving all day and are taking a walk in the late afternoon or evening, you can probably forgo the 5-minute warm-up. Be sure to stretch after you walk.

Wednesday

warm-up: 5 to 10 minutes light stretching

20 to 30 minutes swimming

Take it easy at first if you haven't been swimming in a while. Swim at a moderate pace as continuously as possible. If your arms get tired, go to the shallow end of the pool, and walk. If you are swimming at a health club, there may be water aerobics classes available. Water aerobics is good because it puts very little stress on your joints, which is important for people who haven't done a lot of exercise or who have arthritis or other joint problems.

5 to 10 minutes stretching

Thursday

10- to 15-minute warm-up

25 to 30 minutes weight lifting

Again, you will be performing only 1 set of 12 to 15 repetitions for each exercise. Use light weights. Today you will be working your legs, so your warm-up stretching should focus more on your lower body.

- squats
- leg extensions
- leg curls
- calf raises
- leg abductions (spreading your legs apart in a V)
- leg adductions (starting with your legs in a V and closing your legs)
- lunges (without weights; don't extend your knees past your toes)

5- to 10-minute cooldown (lots of leg stretches)

Friday

10- to 15-minute warm-up

20 to 30 minutes walking (moderate to brisk pace)

You should be able to carry on a conversation while walking.

5- to 10-minute cooldown

Saturday/Sunday

Play. Do anything you want. Gardening, shopping at the mall, playing basketball, hunting, taking a leisurely bike ride—all of these are good activities. Eat a lot of food. On one of these days, don't do anything physical for most of the day. Watch a movie, read a book, play music, get a massage, and get adequate sleep. Be sure to do some stretching during the day and before going to bed.

WEEK 2

This week you will be lifting moderately heavy weight—no more than 60 percent of your maximum weight for each exercise. You will do 2 sets of 8 to 12 repetitions per exercise. It's more important to focus on maintaining good form as opposed to lifting very heavy weights or doing a lot of sets and repetitions.

Monday

warm-up

25 to 30 minutes weight lifting (full body routine)

- inclined bench presses (head higher than feet)
- lat pull-downs (hold bar with palms facing away from you; pull down in front of your face)
- lateral shoulder raises (hold dumbbells and pretend you're a bird flapping your wings)
- sit-ups
- back extensions
- squats
- leg curls
- calf raises

5- to 10-minutes stretching (cooldown)

Tuesday

warm-up

30 minutes walking (moderate to brisk pace)

15 minutes stretching

Wednesday

warm-up

30 to 35 minutes weight lifting (upper body; use dumbbells for exercises requiring weights)

- inclined chest presses
- dumbbell flys
- shoulder presses
- rear deltoid raises (sit on bench; lower chest to knees; begin with hands holding dumbbells at outer thighs; raise dumbbells parallel to ground with arms bent; you should feel the stress on your rear shoulder muscles)
- front deltoid raises (stand with dumbbells held at your sides; raise them in front of you with arms slightly bent; works the front shoulder muscles)
- skull busters (lie back on bench with knees bent and feet on bench; place dumbbells in front of your forehead with the back of your hands facing you; lift dumbbells, stopping at a 90-degree angle from the start position; works your triceps)
- bicep curls
- leg raises (as many as you can do in 1 set)
- abdominal crunches (as many as you can do in 1 set)
- back extensions (as many as you can do in 1 set)
- pull-ups (palms to bar; as many as you can do in 1 set)

cooldown

Thursday

warm-up

15 minutes riding stationary bike or walking (moderate to brisk pace)

20 minutes playing basketball (or another game of your choice: tennis, handball, etc.)

cooldown

Friday

warm-up

25 to 30 minutes weight lifting (lower body)

- squats
- leg extensions
- leg curls
- calf raises
- leg abductions (spreading your legs apart in a **V**)
- leg adductions (starting with your legs in a **V** and closing your legs)
- lunges (without weights; don't extend your knees past your toes)

5- to 10-minute cooldown (lots of leg stretches)

Saturday

30 minutes walking (slow to moderate pace)

1 to 2 hours yard work or gardening

1-hour visit to the mall

Sunday

rest

WEEK 3

This week you will lift weights on 4 days, focusing on a specific part of the body on the first 3 days and doing a full-body routine on the fourth day. Except for the fourth day, your workouts will be shorter than in the previous weeks. Try to lift 75 percent of your maximum weight for each exercise. Do 3 sets of each exercise unless otherwise indicated. Each set should include as many repetitions as possible. Focus on maintaining good form. Don't sacrifice form in exchange for more repetitions. And don't worry if your third set includes a small number of repetitions. The point is to work the muscles to exhaustion. Rest no more than 30 seconds between each set and 1 minute between each exercise. On nonlifting days, you will walk at a slow to moderate pace for 20 to 30 minutes.

Monday
warm-up
20 to 25 minutes weight lifting
- pull-ups (use a pull-up assist machine if one is necessary and available)
- seated rows
- lat pull-downs
- rear deltoid raises
- back extensions
- seated tricep dips
cooldown

Tuesday
warm-up
20 to 25 minutes weight lifting
- bench presses
- butterfly chest presses
- shoulder presses
- lateral shoulder raises
- abdominal crunches (3 sets; head facing straight ahead, to the right and to the left)
- bicep curls
- wrist curls (palms facing toward and away; works front and back of forearms)
cooldown

Wednesday
warm-up
20 to 25 minutes weight lifting

- squats
- leg extensions
- leg curls
- leg presses
- calf raises
- lunges (with weight bar or light dumbbells; be careful not to extend your knees past your toes when stepping forward)

cooldown

Thursday

30 minutes walking (moderate to brisk pace)
15 minutes stretching

Friday

warm-up

- inclined bench presses (head higher than feet)
- lat pull-downs (hold bar with palms facing away from you; pull down in front of your face)
- lateral shoulder raises (hold dumbbells and pretend you're a bird flapping your wings)
- sit-ups
- back extensions
- squats
- leg curls
- calf raises

10 to 15 minutes stretching (cooldown)

Saturday

30 minutes walking
10 to 15 minutes stretching

Sunday
Rest

WEEK 4

This week you will lift weights only 3 days. You'll repeat previous routines used for the upper and lower parts of your body. Again attempt no more than 75 percent of your maximum weight for each exercise. Try to increase the number of repetitions you perform in every set over last week's performance. But don't sacrifice good form for more reps. For each weight lifting exercise, do 3 sets.

Monday
warm-up
20 to 25 minutes weight lifting
- bench presses
- butterfly chest presses
- shoulder presses
- lateral shoulder raises
- abdominal crunches (3 sets; head facing straight ahead, to the right and to the left)
- bicep curls
- wrist curls (palms facing toward and away; works front and back of forearms)

cool down

Tuesday
warm-up
choose an aerobic activity: swimming, walking, stationary biking, rowing machine, aerobics class
cooldown

Wednesday

warm-up

20 to 25 minutes weight lifting

- squats
- leg extensions
- leg curls
- leg presses
- calf raises
- lunges (with weight bar or light dumbbells; be careful not to extend your knees past your toes when stepping forward)

cooldown

Thursday

warm-up

choose an aerobic activity

cooldown

Friday

warm-up

20 to 25 minutes weight lifting

- pull-ups (use a pull-up assist machine if one is necessary and available)
- seated rows
- lat pull-downs
- rear deltoid raises
- back extensions
- seated tricep dips

cooldown

Saturday

warm-up

choose a semi-aerobic activity: basketball, tennis, racquetball, kickboxing class, yard work, leisure bike riding, touch football, etc.

Sunday

20 minutes stretching (while in front of television)

rest

WEEK 5

Week 5 will be fairly easy. The idea is to give your body a well-deserved rest. Do things you enjoy, and add some extra physical activity into your daily routine (i.e., carry your own groceries, take the stairs instead of the elevator, etc.). Don't cut back on food even though you're not exercising as much this week. You won't gain body fat if you're eating according to the NeanderThin program.

Monday

10 minutes stretching
10 minutes walking
1 set push-ups
1 set pull-ups
1 set sit-ups
1 set back extensions
10 minutes light stretching

Tuesday

rest

Wednesday

rest

Thursday

warm-up

15 to 20 minutes weight lifting (full body routine; 1 set of each exercise using light weight)

- inclined bench presses (head higher than feet)
- lat pull-downs (hold bar with palms facing away from you; pull down in front of your face)
- lateral shoulder raises (hold dumbbells and pretend you're a bird flapping your wings)
- sit-ups
- back extensions
- squats
- leg curls
- calf raises

Friday

20 minutes walking

15 to 20 minutes stretching

Saturday/Sunday

rest, stretching, and playing

During Week 6 start the 5-week cycle over again. Change it if you want. Tailor the cycle to fit your personal fitness goals. Every 3 or 4 months, go a week or so without lifting weights at all. The point of this kind of workout regimen is to keep it somewhat regular but not rigid or static. Your body will thrive on a semirandom, semistructured approach to exercise. You can customize your "routine" to include any physical activity you enjoy. One or two hours of serious gardening can replace a full-body weight lifting workout. Just make sure that your program isn't too random. Don't go 3 or 4 weeks without at least some moderate exercise. Even serious athletes can benefit from a "chaotic" approach to exercise. If you're an athlete, the demands of your sport will dictate the kinds of exercises (as well as their intensity) you need to work on primarily.

If you are unfamiliar with the world of weight lifting, it's worth the cost of a few sessions with a personal trainer to learn how to use the machines at your local health club or gym. Once you know how to use the machines, you can make up a weight training program that suits your needs.

One very important thing to keep in mind is that as we get older we tend to lose flexibility. Weight lifting will help you maintain strong bones and muscles. Aerobic exercise will help keep your heart, lungs, and entire circulatory system strong. But to stay flexible, you will need to do some stretching at least every other day. It's best to stretch more intensely after a moderate or intense workout, because your muscles are more limber and pliable after exercise. If you stretch before exercising, stretch lightly and gently. A good book on stretching or a personal trainer can help you to create a simple, effective stretching program. Better yet, join a yoga class. Whatever the approach, for those of us who spend a lot of time indoors, in front of computers and televisions or on the phone—i.e., on our butts—maintaining good flexibility through regular stretching is important.

In this fast-paced world of ours, remember that quality exercise need not take a long time. You should be able to complete a good workout within 30 to 50 minutes. By incorporating more physical activity (taking stairs instead of elevators, parking farther away from the store, etc.) into your daily routine, eating a natural diet, and exercising in a semistructured way, you will find that physical fitness is not that hard to achieve and maintain. You will probably discover that you have no need for extraordinarily complex or expensive exercise routines or equipment.

In nature, being out of shape is a terminal illness. But even if you never have to chase a mastodon over a cliff or wrestle a saber-toothed tiger, as a hunter-gatherer you will find increased strength and stamina beneficial in your everyday life. By eating a natural diet and following natural patterns of physical exertion, you will also find that good muscle tone, endurance, strength, and flexibility come naturally. By keeping your routine convenient, varied, and filled with activities you enjoy, you'll find it easy to make exercise a regular part of your life.

CHAPTER ELEVEN

What to Expect from Following NeanderThin

Any diet, no matter how natural, will require some adjustment, not only socially but also in the body's ability to process the new mix of nutrients being fed to it. A lifetime of eating unnatural foods requires the body to produce large amounts of digestive enzymes that a more natural diet would require only in small amounts. These enzymes are necessary to process large amounts of complex carbohydrates. The body must learn to suppress these enzymes. The overproduction of these enzymes has also inhibited production of other enzymes used to digest natural foods, and the body must now start producing these enzymes to process larger amounts of more natural foods such as meats and fats. As a result, large meals may give you a feeling of heaviness when this change is first undertaken. This feeling will pass quickly as the body adjusts to a more natural balance.

When you change what goes in the body, what comes out changes as well. Your bowel movements will change in both regularity and substance. Similar differences are found in the appearance of coyote scat and the feces left by domestic dogs fed commercial foods. Natural fecal matter has a looser consistency than that resulting from the incomplete digestion of unnatural foods. Natural foods are also processed faster and eliminated more quickly. Don't mistake the increase in frequency and looseness for diarrhea. Soon the body will adjust and increased regularity will follow.

As your body learns to digest and eliminate natural foods more quickly, you will experience a strong increase in appetite. This increased desire for food is often quite disconcerting to the new hunter-gatherer, although it is entirely natural and even desirable. This new hunger will make the new foods you are eating that much more satisfying. Preventing hunger is easy—just eat! Hunger will slow the metabolism as it forces the body to put more energy into making fat, so avoid hunger whenever possible. If it feels like you're eating all the time, you're well on your way to reaching your goals.

Don't mistake increased hunger for cravings. Cravings for forbidden foods are to be expected as all of these unnatural substances produce chemical addictions. These addictions are identical to the complex-carbohydrate cravings of the alcoholic or heroin addict. Whether the source is a drug or a bagel, the endorphins (morphine-like substances) produced by the brain are the same, and it is these unnatural levels of endorphins that we crave. The feelings of fullness, well-being, and tranquility that are produced by these chemicals are most noticeable after a full agricultural feast such as Thanksgiving. You feel sleepy and lethargic—ready to watch football. In contrast, a large hunter-gather meal leaves you feeling energetic and ready to participate in a game of your own.

As with any addiction, withdrawal symptoms are to be expected. These may include nervousness, irritability, insomnia, irregular bowel movements, and, most commonly, cravings for the forbidden substances. How you deal with cravings will have a major impact on your ability to achieve the hunter-gather lifestyle.

Controlling Your Cravings

The easiest way to eliminate cravings is to eliminate the offending substances completely. Just as the alcoholic must never take a drink, so must the hunter-gatherer eliminate even the smallest amount of forbidden fruit. If you religiously avoid the forbidden fruit, your cravings will soon subside completely. The smallest act of cheating may result in a high level of craving. Indeed, 1 potato chip can make you crave an entire bag (for about a week).

As cravings are stimulated by taste, even sugar substitutes such as aspartame or cyclamates may produce cravings of their own. Avoiding sugar-free foods completely will be far easier than trying to use them to wean yourself from sweets or sodas. Carbonated water is often a good substitute for those who crave sodas, but beware of unnaturally sweetened varieties masquerading as natural.

Cravings can be controlled through the use of high-fat snack foods. Eating pemmican, nuts, bacon, or pork rinds (low salt preferred) will greatly reduce your craving for sweets and provide an energy boost as well.

Eating Between Meals

Given these cravings and increasing hunger, proper snacking is vital to maintaining the NeanderThin lifestyle. The best way to ensure availability of proper snacks is to always carry a supply with you. Nuts, fruits, and dried meats require no refrigeration, and you can easily carry them in a pocket, purse, or glove compartment. Carrying water is also a good idea as, often, only colas and beer are available at public events.

Eating between meals is encouraged, but it is also helpful to increase the size of each meal. People in general, but especially former dieters, are hesitant at first to eat the increased portions required to satisfy NeanderThin needs. Some (especially women in our repressive society) may be embarrassed and worry that others may perceive them as overeating. Have faith that as your weight decreases, those looks of disapproval will change to looks of amazement. It is important to remember to prepare meals with your new appetite in mind. Try to make more than you think you need. Having leftovers will provide a feeling of security as well as late-night snacks.

The Results Speak for Themselves

Of course, all of these adjustments will become easier as you see the results of the NeanderThin program. Any inconvenience will be offset by these results, and lifestyle changes will become second nature in a short time. For most people the benefits will be so great as to make the idea of returning to an agricultural diet unthinkable.

The most noticeable of these benefits, in most cases, is weight loss. This weight loss may be most dramatic in the initial adjustment period. Losing several pounds per week is not unusual. During this period it is very important to drink lots of water to forestall the side effects of burning large amounts of body fats in a process called *ketosis.*

Ketosis is a condition in which your body converts from burning carbohydrate-based fuel to using your stored fat reserves for energy. Removing most or all carbohydrate from your diet sparks the ketogenic process. Fat is broken down into ketones, which are used by brain cells, and free fatty acids, used by the body for muscular activity. Excess ketones produced by the fat-burning process are excreted in the breath and urine. By increasing liquid intake you make sure they come out through the urine, and not the breath, where they can produce an unpleasant odor.

If you add a significant number of carbohydrates to your diet, weight loss may slow or even stall completely. A very small amount of cheating can also produce such an episode. Should this occur, weight loss can be resumed by forcing the body to start producing ketones again. This can be accomplished by eliminating all carbohydrates (fruits and vegetables) completely. By becoming completely carnivorous for a period of 24 to 48 hours, the body will be forced to begin burning its stored fat. You can monitor your body's progression into a state of ketosis by using test strips (available at any drugstore) to detect the presence of ketones in your urine.

A Word About Ketosis

For the average person there is nothing inherently dangerous about ketosis. Many hunter-gatherers live in a state of ketosis almost year-round. Persons with Type 1 insulin-dependent diabetes are, however, advised to consult a physician before undertaking a low-carbohydrate, ketogenic diet (see Eades, Bernstein, and Atkins in the Bibliography).

It is not necessary to maintain the state of ketosis produced by an exclusive meat and fat diet. As you reach a state of ketosis, add small amounts of vegetable foods over the next few days until weight loss slows again and maintain carbohydrates at that level. As your metabolism increases you can increase the vegetable portion again to taste.

Increased Energy, Increased Activity, Increased Weight Loss

Increased physical activity will also help you to accelerate weight loss. Increasing physical activity is made easier by the increase in metabolic rate inherent in this program. Your metabolism increases because the body begins to spend less of its energy resources on immune responses to alien proteins in food. This energy is now available for use in metabolic processes such as digestion, tissue regeneration, and muscle development.

At first this new energy may feel somewhat uncomfortable. It may express itself in the form of restlessness, nervousness, or insomnia. The solution is to increase your physical activity to match the increase in your metabolic rate. (See Chapter 10 for a full, five-week fitness and activity plan). As you increase the amount of physical activity in your life, this discomfort will be eliminated. It will be replaced by the sense of calm and well being associated with physical exertion, as opposed to the worn-out feeling often caused by stress on the immune system.

A Boost to Your Immune System

As less of your body's energy is being consumed by immunological responses to alien proteins, more of your immune system resources are available to combat disease not attributable to dietary practices. In cultures that survive on technology-dependent foods exclusively (i.e., vegetarian cultures), diseases such as measles, mumps, and influenza—considered minor in industrialized countries—result in extremely high mortality rates. In contrast, the hunter-gatherer experiences much milder colds, influenza, mononucleosis, and yeast infections. Many people also notice that minor cuts and abrasions heal much faster.

Allergic reactions will also be reduced, but for a different reason. These particular immune reactions include itchy and watery eyes, runny nose, asthma, sneezing, hives, dry skin, headaches, lethargy, and fluid retention. All of these reactions are considered threshold phenomena; that is, until exposure to the allergen involved reaches a certain level, there is no response. But once that level is reached, the response is immediate and total. When your diet regularly exposes you to foreign proteins, the baseline of response is much closer to this threshold, resulting in allergic attacks to much smaller amounts of allergens than would affect a hunter-gatherer. From the evolutionary standpoint, it would be very difficult to survive hay fever attacks that affect your senses of sight, hearing, and smell if you made your living as a hunter.

In conclusion, it should be noted that as dramatic as the results of NeanderThin are, the consequences of quitting are even more dramatic. Whether you decide to quit entirely or even partially, you will probably gain weight faster than before. Because your immune system is stronger on the NeanderThin diet, your body's immune response to technology-dependent foods will be much stronger after adopting the diet. The other health benefits that go along with the NeanderThin program will disappear as well. If you have been following the program religiously, cheating will often result in illness. The nausea, lethargy, intestinal gas, constipation, fluid retention, and so on that will accompany an episode of cheating can serve as excellent reinforcement against cheating or quitting. If it feels bad, don't do it. The best defense against cheating is to eat a varied diet that is rich in flavor. If you regularly eat your fill of good food and avoid hunger, you are much less likely to give in to the temptations prohibited by NeanderThin. Achieving this level of dietary satisfaction is simple, as you will see in the following chapter.

CHAPTER TWELVE

Recipes, Menu Suggestions, and a Food Diary

There are a wide variety of low-carbohydrate recipe books available, such as *Dr. Atkin's Quick and Easy New Diet Cookbook* and *The Low-Carb Cookbook,* which contain many recipes that are NeanderThin friendly. If you concentrate on cooking foods containing only ingredients on the NeanderThin "Do Eat" list, you can also find appropriate recipes in general cookbooks, such as *The Nika Hazelton Way with Vegetables, Ten Talents Cookbook,* and the *Three Rivers Cookbook* series. On the Internet, you'll find that www.paleofood.com offers an extensive list of menu and recipe suggestions.

Many of the recipes in this chapter have been adapted from those sent in by readers following the NeanderThin eating plan. Others I have created or adapted from various sources and turned into personal favorites.

After adopting the NeanderThin program, you will most likely find that your life in the kitchen is simplified. Your food preparation time will be reduced as will the amount of waste that you generate. You might want to start a compost pile to accommodate the scraps from the increased amount of fresh, raw foods you will be eating.

Most of the recipes that follow have a low-carbohydrate content.

Stay away from the high-carb recipes until you have reached your desired body weight. If you have cholesterol or blood sugar problems, you will also want to avoid the higher-carb recipes.

RECIPES

Breakfast

Spinach, Mushroom, and Bacon Frittata

For those who like quiche, the Italian frittata is a wonderful substitute.

INGREDIENTS:
½ pound fresh raw spinach
1 pound fresh mushrooms
⅓ cup olive oil
3 to 4 scallions, thinly sliced
2 cloves garlic
½ teaspoon salt
½ teaspoon freshly ground black pepper
8 eggs, at room temperature
4 to 6 slices crisply cooked bacon (uncured), crumbled

1. Carefully wash spinach, and remove stems. Place in a colander to drain. Slice mushrooms thinly.

2. In a 12-inch omelet pan, or a large skillet with sloping sides, heat 2 tablespoons of the olive oil over medium-low heat. Add the scallions and the garlic and sauté until they have softened.

3. Add the sliced mushrooms, salt, and pepper. Turn the heat to medium, and sauté the mushrooms until they give up their liquid and it evaporates. Remove the pan from the heat to cool.

4. In a large mixing bowl, beat the eggs until they are light. Finely chop the drained spinach, and add it to the eggs, then add the cooled mushroom mixture and the bacon. Stir to blend. Preheat your oven's broiler.

5. Wipe the omelet pan clean with a paper towel, place it back on the stove over medium-high heat, and add the remaining olive oil. When the oil is hot, pour in the egg mixture. Quickly give the pan a few vigorous shakes back and forth across the burner surface to make sure the frittata does not stick; then immediately turn the heat to very low to avoid burning the bottom. Let cook for 20 minutes (more or less) without stirring.

6. When the egg mixture is set, but the top is still a little runny, remove the frittata from the stove and place it under the broiler for 1 to 2 minutes until the eggs have just set, but do not brown the top.

7. With the aid of a spatula, slide the frittata onto a serving platter and slice into wedges. The flavors of the vegetables will be more pronounced if you serve the frittata at room temperature.

Serves 2 to 4

Fried Apples and Bacon

INGREDIENTS:

½ pound bacon (preferably uncured)

3 or 4 apples

1. Fry bacon. Pat dry with paper towel, and retain grease in frying pan.

2. Chop apples into bite-size pieces. Peel apples before chopping (optional).

3. Fry apples in hot bacon grease. The longer you fry apples, the softer their consistency.

4. When apples are done, remove from pan and pat dry with a paper towel.

5. Crumble bacon, toss with apples, and serve.

Serves 2 to 4

Vegetable Juice Omelet

INGREDIENTS:

1 cup chopped fresh spinach
4 green onions, chopped
1 clove fresh garlic, chopped
½ cup mushrooms
3 eggs
¼ cup vegetable juice (V8, etc.)
Salt, pepper, cayenne pepper to taste

1. Sauté chopped vegetables in hot olive oil heated on medium to high.

2. Beat eggs in a separate bowl. Then mix eggs with vegetable juice and seasonings.

3. Pour egg mixture into pan and cook until omelet is golden brown on bottom (raise omelet with fork or spatula to check color).

4. Flip omelet and cook until other side is golden brown.

5. Garnish with sweet pepper, tomato slices, chopped cilantro, or parsley, as desired.

Serves 1

Nut Milk

INGREDIENTS:

1 cup almonds
Apple juice
½ teaspoon honey (optional)
Purified water

1. Pour almonds into a bowl or glass and add enough apple juice to cover. Soak overnight.
2. Pour Almonds and apple juice into blender. Add honey (if used) and 5 to 6 ounces of water and blend until mixture is liquefied.

Serves 1 or 2

Applesauce

Don't eat a lot of applesauce if you need to avoid large amounts of carbohydrates. Make applesauce an occasional treat.

INGREDIENTS:

8 apples (golden delicious, red delicious, etc.)
⅓ cup honey
2 to 3 tablespoons fresh lemon juice to taste (lemon juice is a
    good preservative)

1. Peel apples, remove cores, slice into quarters, and place in blender.
2. Add honey and lemon juice to blender.
3. Blend until mixture is smooth (high blender setting).
4. Keep refrigerated. Use within 1 or 2 days.

Makes 4 to 5 servings

Green Onions and Eggs

INGREDIENTS:

2 bunches wild green onions
3 tablespoons bacon fat (or 4 tablespoons olive oil); use more fat
   or oil if using jumbo eggs
8 large eggs
Salt and pepper to taste
¼ cup water

1. Wash onions. Slice off tips and discard. Dice remaining tops and stems.

2. Heat bacon fat (or olive oil) in a large, heavy skillet over medium heat.

3. Add onions to skillet. Mix onions with fat or oil until completely coated.

4. Cover skillet, lower heat, and let cook for 1 or 2 minutes.

5. While waiting, crack eggs and place into a bowl. Beat until whites and yolks are thoroughly mixed.

6. Uncover skillet. Add seasonings and water. Cover again and let cook for another 1 or 2 minutes. (For more tender onions, cook a few minutes longer and add more water as necessary.)

7. Remove skillet lid and pour in eggs. Add more seasonings if desired. Stir mixture until eggs are no longer runny.

8. Spoon eggs and onions onto a plate and serve hot. Try adding salsa to the eggs for additional flavor.

Serves 2 to 3 (depending on size of eggs)

NOTE: If you like, you may substitute garlic, young leeks, chives, or a combination for 1 onion bunch.

Puffy Omelet

INGREDIENTS:

4 eggs, separated
¼ cup water
¼ teaspoon salt
⅛ teaspoon pepper
1½ tablespoons bacon fat (enough bacon fat, or olive oil, to thickly coat omelet pan)

1. Beat egg whites, water, and salt with a mixer in a small bowl until mixture is stiff but not dry.
2. Separately beat egg yolks and pepper until mixture is thick.
3. Preheat oven to 325 degrees.
4. Heat fat in omelet pan (or cast-iron skillet). Pan should be just hot enough to make a drop of water sizzle on contact.
5. Pour contents of both bowls into skillet. Stir to combine and level mixture.
6. Lower heat and cook on low heat until puffy and light brown on the bottom (use a spatula to raise omelet and check color).
7. Place omelet in oven for approximately 15 minutes.
8. Take omelet out of oven. Tilt the skillet or pan and slide spatula under omelet. Slide the omelet from the pan onto a plate, then fold in half. Serve hot.

Serves 1

Chilis, Soups, and Stews

Chili

This legendary food, named "the state dish of Texas" by the Texas legislature, has been a source of many debates, both as to the origin and the correct ingredients. It has been said by some of the most respected figures in the chili world that "anyone who would put beans in chili doesn't know beans about chili." The following recipe is a "no frills" version. Included are a couple of the most common variations for the more adventurous who would "fly in the face" of Texas tradition.

INGREDIENTS:
2 ounces animal fat (beef suet or uncured bacon)
2 pounds coarsely ground beef
½ cup finely chopped onion
2 cloves garlic, minced
2 tablespoons chili powder, or more if desired
½ teaspoon ground cumin
⅛ teaspoon dried oregano (optional)
Salt to taste

1. In a large skillet (preferably cast-iron), render fat over medium heat and remove rinds. Add ground beef to skillet and cook until just brown. Add onion and garlic.

2. Add chili powder, cumin, and oregano, and mix well. Add salt conservatively.

3. Reduce heat to low and let simmer for at least 2 hours. The texture and flavor will change greatly as all of the ingredients blend together.

4. Add water as needed during cooking, keeping in mind that the final product should be somewhat thick.

Serves 3 to 6

VARIATIONS: Instead of adding water if it is needed, add tomato juice or pureed tomatoes. Chopped mushrooms and green peppers also make great additions.

Green Chili Stew

INGREDIENTS:
2 dozen green chile peppers (hot, mild, jalapeño, whatever you
   prefer, preferably fresh)
2-pound pork loin
2 tablespoons olive oil
3 cloves garlic, minced
½ teaspoon cumin
2 large onions, finely chopped
3 cups stewed tomatoes
2 cups water
2 teaspoons salt

1. If chile peppers are fresh, roast, then place in a paper bag to loosen peels, and after removing all peels, ribs, seeds, and tops, cut peppers into 1-inch slices.
2. Cut pork into bite-size pieces.
3. Heat olive oil in a large pot, and add pork.
4. When pork is fully cooked (no pink meat or juices), add remaining ingredients, and allow mixture to cook at medium-low heat for 1 hour until ingredients combine into a thick stew.
5. Season to taste, and serve hot for best results.

Serves 4 to 6

Chicken Soup

Nothing is more filling or warming on a cold winter day than a bowl of chicken soup.

INGREDIENTS:

1 whole deboned precooked chicken with giblets
4 stalks celery, chopped
2 large carrots, chopped
1 onion, chopped
½ teaspoon poultry seasoning

1. In a large pot add chicken and giblets, chopped vegetables, and poultry seasoning.
2. Add enough water to cover everything.
3. Bring to a boil.
4. Let simmer for 15 minutes.
5. Serve hot.

Serves 4 to 6 (depending on size of chicken)

Beef Soup

Favored by Arctic explorers for ease of preparation and as a source of energy and warmth.

INGREDIENTS:

1 cup water
2 tablespoons hamburger or 1 tablespoon Pemmican (page 147)

1. Bring water to a boil.
2. Add hamburger or pemmican and stir until water boils again.
3. Serve hot.

Serves 1

Leftover Soup

This recipe is a catchall for leftovers that may be cluttering your refrigerator.

INGREDIENTS:

Chopped leftover meats
Chopped leftover vegetables
Olive oil
Seasonings to taste

1. Add leftover chicken, turkey, roast beef, or other meat to a soup pot.
2. Add leftover celery, carrots, mushrooms, onions, etc., to the meat.
3. Cover meat and vegetables with water.
4. Add 3 or 4 tablespoons of olive oil and any seasonings you may want (salt, pepper, poultry seasoning, etc.)
5. Bring soup to a boil and turn down heat. Let soup simmer for 20 minutes or so.
6. Serve hot.

*Number of servings depends on amounts of
meat, vegetables, and water*

Roman Egg Drop Soup

INGREDIENTS:

4 cups chicken broth
2 cups chopped washed fresh spinach
2 eggs, beaten

1 tablespoon grated lemon rind
Salt and pepper to taste

1. Bring broth to a boil, add spinach, and boil gently on high for several minutes.
2. Mix eggs, lemon rind, salt, and pepper.
3. Lower heat, stir in egg mixture, and cook for a minute or so until eggs set.

Serves 3

Appetizers

Deviled Eggs

Ray's secret weapon.

INGREDIENTS:
8 hard-boiled eggs (chilled)
3 tablespoons NeanderThin Mayonnaise (page 132)
¼ teaspoon dry mustard
6 slices bacon (uncured), fried and crumbled
Salt to taste

1. Slice eggs lengthwise. Separate yolks and whites, placing yolks in a bowl.
2. Combine mayonnaise, mustard, bacon, and salt with yolks. Blend until mixture takes on a smooth consistency.
3. Spoon mixture into egg whites. Cover and chill again if eggs are not to be eaten immediately.

Serves 4 to 8

Shrimp Cocktail

INGREDIENTS:

1 pound shrimp
7 tablespoons chili sauce (or NeanderThin Barbecue Sauce,
    page 135)
2 tablespoons lemon juice
Pinch of salt
¼ teaspoon grated onion
⅔ cup celery, chopped finely
2 cups salad greens (iceberg or romaine lettuce)
Lemon slices

1. Boil shrimp. Then peel them and remove tails. Refrigerate in a covered bowl.
2. Make cocktail sauce in a separate bowl by mixing chili (or NeanderThin Barbecue) sauce, lemon juice, salt, and onion.
3. Add celery to shrimp and mix.
4. Arrange beds of salad greens in wide-mouth wineglasses.
5. Add shrimp mixture to glasses, spoon cocktail sauce onto shrimp mixture, and add two to three lemon slices for garnish.
6. Serve cold for best results.

Serves 4 to 5 depending on size of glasses

Cold Shrimp-Stuffed Avocados

INGREDIENTS:

3 large avocados
Juice of 1 lemon
1 pound cooked shelled shrimp (minus 6 whole shrimp reserved
    for garnish), coarsely chopped

1 pound fresh hot chile pepper (peeled, seeded, washed, and
  chopped fine)
1 hard-cooked egg, chopped
2 dozen pitted green or black olives
⅓ cup NeanderThin Mayonnaise (page 132)
Salt and pepper
3 tablespoons fresh coriander or parsley leaves, minced

1. Slice avocados in half (lengthwise), remove the pits, and
spoon out the flesh. Place avocado pieces in a bowl.

2. Splash avocado shells and pieces with lemon juice to prevent
oxidation (darkening of the flesh). Set shells aside (don't throw
shells away!).

3. Use a fork to mash the avocado. Add shrimp, hot pepper, egg,
and olives to the flesh, mixing thoroughly. Add mayonnaise while
stirring the mixture.

4. Add salt and pepper to taste.

5. Spoon the mixture into the avocado shells. Garnish each shell
with a whole shrimp and a sprinkle of coriander or parsley and a
splash of lemon juice.

6. Serve immediately for best results.

Serves 3 to 6

Nut Sushi

Visit a health food store or an imported food market to purchase the dried seaweed called for in this recipe.

INGREDIENTS:

1 cup nuts (pine nuts, almonds, hazelnuts, macadamias, chestnuts, etc.)
⅓ cup fresh cilantro or parsley
½ cup onion, diced
2 large avocados, sliced
1 tomato, diced
Juice of 1 lemon
2 garlic cloves, chopped finely
Dried seaweed strips torn from large sheet (wide, lengthwise strips)

1. Grind nuts into very small crumbs in a meat grinder or food processor.
2. Put ground nuts, cilantro, onion, avocado, tomato, lemon juice, and garlic in a bowl. Mix thoroughly.
3. Spoon mixture onto a seaweed strip and wrap the strip into a ball around the mixture. Pierce with a toothpick to hold the "sushi" wrap together. Repeat until mixture is gone.
4. Refrigerate until ready to eat.

Makes approximately 6 servings depending on size of strips

Nut Pizza

INGREDIENTS:

2 cups nuts (Brazil, macadamias, walnuts, hazelnuts, hickory, etc.)
3 tomatoes, sliced

2 cloves garlic, minced
1 sweet pepper, diced
1 onion, diced
1 cup pine nuts
1 cup sausage, precooked
1 teaspoon oregano

1. Preheat oven to 225 degrees.

2. Grind nuts into crumbs/mush using a blender or a food processor.

3. Steam vegetables for 2 to 3 minutes (except for tomatoes, vegetables should still be crisp when done).

4. Add ground nuts, vegetables, and sausage (in that order) to a baking pan or dish. Sprinkle oregano evenly over pizza.

5. Place pizza into oven for no more than 2 minutes.

6. Remove from oven and garnish with pine nuts or vegetables as desired. Serve warm for best results.

Serves 2 to 4

Salads

Waldorf Salad

This recipe will have a special place in the heart of any John Cleese and Fawlty Towers *fan.*

INGREDIENTS:

3 firm crisp apples (red Delicious, Golden Delicious, or a combination of the two)
1 tablespoon freshly squeezed lemon juice
1 cup cut-up celery, cut crosswise
½ cup coarsely chopped walnuts
½ cup NeanderThin Mayonnaise (page 132)
1½ tablespoons raw unfiltered honey (optional)
Lettuce leaves (optional)

1. Core and quarter apples and cut into ½-inch pieces. Put in a bowl and toss with lemon juice to coat. Add the celery and walnuts. Cover and chill.

2. Blend mayonnaise and apple mixture together (see Note). If desired, serve on a bed of lettuce leaves.

Serves 2 to 3

NOTE: If using honey, blend with mayonnaise at this time.

Simple, Perfect Chicken Salad

A classic made NeanderThin style.

INGREDIENTS:

3 cups cut-up cooled cooked chicken (removed from bones and
cut into bite-size pieces)
1 cup NeanderThin Mayonnaise (page 132)
1 cup finely chopped celery
Salad greens
Optional garnishes include the following: boiled eggs and
parsley; walnut halves and watercress sprigs; or almonds,
green peppers, and Italian parsley

1. Combine chicken, mayonnaise, and celery in a large bowl and
mix well.
2. Serve on a bed of salad greens.

Serves 1 to 2

Tuna Salad with Onion, Avocado, and Egg

*Our tuna salad is made with gourmet-quality tuna
packed in olive oil. Most commercial canned tuna is
packed with either spring water or vegetable oil and contains an ingredient called hydrolyzed vegetable protein,
which is often derived from corn. Such low-grade
canned tunas should be avoided. If you are unable to
find tuna that is not packed using unacceptable methods
and does not contain forbidden substances, try substitut-
ing fresh tuna or even chicken in this recipe instead.*

127

INGREDIENTS:

1 head lettuce, washed, dried, and separated into leaves
Two 7-ounce cans imported Italian tuna, packed in olive oil
    (see Note)
1 cup freshly sliced onion rings
1 cup diced avocado
4 hard-boiled eggs, quartered
2 to 3 tablespoons capers (optional)
½ to ¾ cup A Vinegarless Vinaigrette (page 131)

1. Put greens in a large salad bowl, and place tuna, onion rings, avocado, eggs, and capers on top.
2. Dress with the vinaigrette. Toss and serve.

Serves 2 to 4

NOTE: If imported tuna is unavailable, substitute 14 ounces fresh tuna or chicken. Add approximately ½ cup of olive oil and toss.

NeanderThin Guacamole

Use guacamole as a dip for other snack foods or as a dressing or condiment.

INGREDIENTS:

4 large ripe avocados
4 tablespoons freshly squeezed lemon juice
1 cup minced onion
1 cup chopped fresh tomato
4 sprigs fresh cilantro or parsley
4 small hot chile peppers, minced
4 teaspoons minced garlic
Salt to taste

1. Slice avocados lengthwise, remove pits, and scrape fruit into a bowl.

2. Mash fruit with a fork, add remaining ingredients, and blend thoroughly.

3. Sprinkle extra lemon juice on top of mixture and chill if not to be served immediately.

Serves 4 to 6

Venetian Salad

This is a well-balanced salad, sure to please lovers of Italian food.

INGREDIENTS:

1 head Romaine lettuce, bruised outer leaves removed
1 bunch arugula, stems trimmed
1 green pepper, julienned
1 tomato, cut into wedges
6 mushrooms, thinly sliced
½ cucumber, thinly sliced
½ bunch seedless grapes, halved
¼ cup extra virgin olive oil
Juice of ½ lemon
Salt and freshly ground black pepper to taste

1. Combine vegetables and grapes in a large salad bowl.
2. Add olive oil and lemon juice.
3. Add salt and pepper to taste.
4. Toss gently.

Serves 3 to 4

Slaw

INGREDIENTS:

½ head cabbage
2 carrots
1 onion
1 egg, beaten
1 cup NeanderThin Mayonnaise (see page 132)
1 tablespoon fresh lemon juice
Salt and pepper to taste
1 tablespoon honey (optional)

1. Grate cabbage, carrots, and onion, and mix them in a bowl.
2. Make dressing in a separate bowl by mixing beaten egg, mayonnaise, lemon juice, seasonings, and honey (if used).
3. Add dressing to grated vegetables and mix thoroughly.
4. For best results, chill slaw before serving.

Serves 2 to 3

Salsa Salad

INGREDIENTS:

1 bunch cilantro
5 to 6 Roma tomatoes
1 small yellow or red onion
2 ripe avocados
1 small chile pepper
½ cup whole dulse leaves
2 or 3 whole limes

1. Chop cilantro. Dice tomatoes, onions, and avocados. Dice chili pepper very finely.

2. Add all ingredients in step 1 to a bowl and mix thoroughly.
3. Tear whole dulse leaf into small pieces and add to other ingredients in bowl.
4. Cut limes and squeeze juice onto other ingredients.
5. Toss and refrigerate. Serve cold.

Number of servings varies with use (dressing, dip, etc.)

Dressing, Sauces, and Condiments

A Vinegarless Vinaigrette

In the NeanderThin program, salads must be eaten without conventional condiments such as croutons, cheese, and commercial salad dressings. Many people, however, find the idea of eating a "dry" salad unsavory. So the following is a recipe for a salad dressing that will add a great deal of flavor to any salad while remaining within the NeanderThin dietary guidelines.

INGREDIENTS:
1 clove garlic
3 tablespoons olive oil
1 tablespoon lemon juice
½ teaspoon dry mustard
Salt and freshly ground pepper to taste

1. Crush garlic clove and rub vigorously on bottom of a small mixing bowl. Discard garlic. (If you are a big garlic fan, you may simply mince the clove and put it in bowl.)
2. Add remaining ingredients to bowl and whisk until everything is thoroughly blended.

Enough for 1 large or 2 small servings

NeanderThin Mayonnaise
(made in a blender or food processor)

Mayonnaise is a popular condiment and need not be abandoned by the modern hunter-gatherer. Commercially produced mayonnaise, however, is rife with chemicals and other undesirable ingredients and, for the most part, should be avoided. Homemade mayo, on the other hand, can be eaten without reservation, because all the ingredients used to make it are acceptable by NeanderThin standards.

INGREDIENTS:

1 whole egg, at room temperature (plus 1 yolk for food
   processor)
½ teaspoon dry mustard
¼ teaspoon salt (crushed sea salt is preferable)
¼ teaspoon (preferably freshly ground) white pepper
   (optional)
1½ tablespoons lemon juice (about 1 small lemon; 2 tablespoons
   for food processor)
1 cup light olive oil (plus ½ cup for food processor)

1. Break egg into bowl of your blender or food processor fitted with steel blade (if using processor add additional yolk). Add dry mustard, salt, white pepper, and lemon juice (if using processor, add 2 tablespoons lemon juice). Cover and blend 3 to 5 seconds.

2. With motor still running, remove plastic stopper from the cover of the blender or the pusher from the food processor and begin adding olive oil (if using processor, add additional ½ cup oil) in a slow, steady stream until all of the oil is used. Blend only until mayonnaise is thick.

3. Scrape mayonnaise into a glass container; cover and refrigerate (if the mayonnaise is not to be used up right away). The mayonnaise will keep for 1 week.

Servings depend on use
(dressing, condiment, or recipe ingredient)

Mom's Ketchup

The NeanderThin-approved version of America's favorite condiment. (Submitted by Ray's mom, who, although in her seventies, is a NeanderThin convert and is not to be trifled with!)

INGREDIENTS:
3⅓ pounds tomatoes, sliced
2 medium sliced onions
⅛ clove garlic
Approximately ½ bay leaf (small)
½ red pepper
¼ cup unsweetened juice (select naturally sweeter ones: white grape, pear, or apple)
1 spice bag (see Notes)
½ cup freshly squeezed lemon juice
Cayenne and coarse salt (optional)

1. Boil tomatoes, onions, garlic, bay leaf, and red pepper until they are soft, about 20–30 minutes. Strain them.
2. Add juice to strained ingredients.

3. Add spice bag to mixture, boiling ingredients quickly, stirring frequently until they are reduced to half the quantity. Remove spice bag.

4. Add lemon juice, cayenne, and salt.

5. Boil ketchup for 10 more minutes. Bottle (see Notes) at once in clean jars leaving ¼ to ¾ inch of headroom (see Notes). Cover and freeze immediately. Always refrigerate container of ketchup that is in use.

Servings depend on use

NOTES: The spices can be varied. Try 1 teaspoon of each of the following: allspice, black peppercorns, celery seeds, cloves, and mace, plus ½-inch cinnamon stick. Tie the spices in cheesecloth.

Choose containers (plastic or glass) of a size that your family will use in a week's time. Since there are no preservatives added, the ketchup can spoil once it is defrosted.

Headroom allows for freezer swell.

Salsa

INGREDIENTS:

2 cloves garlic, minced
1 large onion, diced
1 green bell pepper, seeded, diced
3 or 4 jalapeño peppers, tops removed, diced
6 tomatoes, peeled and chopped
1 cup fresh cilantro
Fresh juice of 2 limes
Salt and pepper to taste

1. Combine all ingredients in a bowl and toss.
2. Serve cold for best results. Refrigerate when not in use.

Number of servings depends on use (dip, dressing, etc.)

NeanderThin Barbecue Sauce

The crown jewel of the NeanderThin kitchen.

INGREDIENTS:

2 cloves garlic, minced
2 tablespoons finely chopped onion
2 tablespoons bacon fat
1 teaspoon chili powder, or more to taste
1 teaspoon dried rosemary leaves, crushed
½ teaspoon coriander seeds, finely ground or crushed
1 teaspoon ground ginger
One 6-ounce can tomato paste
½ cup water, or more if needed
6 ounces 100% natural apple juice concentrate
Juice of 1 orange (⅓ to ½ cup, more or less)

1. Sauté garlic and onion in bacon fat over medium-low heat until tender, 5 to 10 minutes.
2. Add chili powder, rosemary, coriander, and ginger.
3. Add all other ingredients and stir until well blended.
4. Cover and simmer over low heat for at least 30 minutes to let flavors blend. If sauce becomes too thick, add more water.

Serves 2 to 4

Pesto

Pesto is a delicious fresh Italian pasta sauce, but it also makes a good sauce for chicken or fish or a dip for vegetables. It will store almost indefinitely in the refrigerator if you put it in a container, pour a small amount of olive oil on top of it, and cover.

INGREDIENTS:

6 tablespoons good-quality extra virgin olive oil
1 cup shelled walnuts (see Notes)
4 cups tightly packed fresh basil
3 tablespoons Italian parsley
Salt and freshly ground black pepper to taste

Place all ingredients in a blender or food processor and blend until just combined.

Servings depend on use

NOTES: If you want a richer sauce, replace up to half of walnuts with pine nuts.

Pesto can also be used to flavor chicken or fish that is baked or grilled. Simply brush a light coat of pesto on meat and cook as usual.

Try adding pesto to any broth-based soup, such as Roman Egg Drop Soup (page 120) recipe. Just add a tablespoon or so at a time until it suits you.

Entrees

Grilled Venison Steaks with Herbs

INGREDIENTS:

¼ cup olive oil
2 tablespoons chopped garlic
2 tablespoons chopped rosemary
2 tablespoons chopped thyme
4 venison steaks (4 ounces each)
Salt and pepper to taste

1. Combine olive oil, garlic, and herbs to make marinade.
2. Put marinade in a dish large enough for steaks. Place steaks in marinade and put dish in refrigerator for 4 hours.
3. Remove dish from refrigerator, pat steaks dry with paper towels, and place steaks on a large plate.
4. Lay venison steaks on grill over hot coals, add salt and pepper to taste, and brush with marinade while steaks cook. The more marinade, the richer the flavor.
5. Cook steaks to desired degree (preferably rare or medium-rare; cooking more than medium-rare is a waste of good meat). Turn steaks at least one time.

Serves 4

Shish Kebab

INGREDIENTS:

1 clove garlic
½ teaspoon basil
½ cup extra virgin olive oil
¼ cup fresh lemon or lime juice
2 pounds cubed lamb (beef, chicken, whole shrimp, etc.)
1 cup fresh pineapple slices
1 cup baby onions
2 green peppers, quartered and seeded
1 cup cherry tomatoes

1. Mash garlic clove into the bottom of a mixing bowl. Add basil, olive oil, and lemon or lime juice to the bowl and mix ingredients well. Place meat cubes in bowl and place bowl in refrigerator for 4 hours.

2. Remove meat cubes from marinade and place on skewers, alternating meat with pineapples, baby onions, green peppers, and tomatoes.

3. Grill over hot coals until meat is done.

Number of servings depends on size of skewers.
This recipe should serve at least 4.

Fried Chicken

Believe it or not.

INGREDIENTS:

2½ cups olive oil
5 or 6 eggs

Salt and pepper to taste
1½ cups water
8 uncooked chicken drumsticks
4 cups arrowroot or pecan flour (from health food store)

1. Pour olive oil into a deep frying pan and warm over medium heat.
2. Mix eggs, seasonings, and water in a mixing bowl. Mixture should have the consistency of pancake batter. Add water and flour as necessary.
3. Coat raw chicken pieces in egg mixture by dipping pieces into the bowl.
4. Pour flour into a separate bowl. Cover chicken pieces with the flour by rolling each piece through the flour bowl.
5. Place chicken in frying pan. Chicken is done when the flour coating is crunchy and the meat is white (no pink meat or juices revealed when cutting into chicken). Add oil to pan if too much oil absorbed to finish cooking all pieces.

Serves 2 to 4

Baked Fish

INGREDIENTS:
1 whole fish (trout, bass, halibut, salmon, etc.)
Olive oil
Salt and pepper
Thyme
Rosemary
Lemon slices
Tomato slices

1. Preheat oven to 350 degrees.

2. Remove head and tail of fish. Make one long cut down center of fish belly, removing innards and bones.

3. Fill hollow cavity with olive oil and close.

4. Mix salt and herbs in a bowl and rub mixture onto fish.

5. Wrap fish in parchment paper and put fish in a baking dish.

6. Allow to bake in oven until fish is flaky (approximately 15 minutes).

7. Garnish with lemon and tomato slices, and serve hot.

Serves 1 or 2 depending on size of fish

Scampi

INGREDIENTS:

1 pound shrimp

4 cloves garlic

½ cup lemon juice

½ to 1 cup extra virgin olive oil

½ tablespoon salt

¼ teaspoon pepper

½ teaspoon oregano

1. Peel shrimp and remove tails. Chill in a bowl.

2. Mash garlic cloves in a mixing bowl and add remaining ingredients.

3. Pour the marinade over the shrimp and refrigerate for 3 or 4 hours.

4. Steam shrimp for 20 to 30 minutes (medium-high heat).

5. Serve hot.

Serves 2 to 4

Pepper Steak

INGREDIENTS:

1 large onion
1 large sweet pepper (green, red, or yellow)
1 pound round steak (½ inch thick)
2 tablespoons olive oil
Salt, pepper, garlic powder to taste
¼ cup water

1. Dice onion and green pepper.
2. Slice beef in long thin strips. (Your butcher can do this for you using an industrial meat slicer.) Then cut each strip into smaller sections.
3. Put olive oil in a deep skillet over medium-high heat. Brown meat for 1 minute.
4. Add pepper, salt, and garlic powder to taste. Also add water, onions, and green pepper.
5. Stir ingredients for 4 or 5 minutes.
6. Serve hot.

Serves 2 to 4

Grilled Chicken with Salsa

INGREDIENTS:

1 cup Salsa (page 135)
4 boneless skinless chicken breasts

1. Pour salsa into a bowl or large plastic freezer bag. Add chicken and refrigerate. Allow to marinate for 4 or 5 hours.
2. Grill chicken breasts over hot coals (no flame).

3. Brush chicken with fresh salsa while grilling. Don't use the marinade, as it contains raw chicken juices.

4. Chicken is done when meat is white throughout the breast (no pink flesh or juices). Pierce chicken with a fork or knife to check. Cooking time should be 15 to 20 minutes.

Serves 2 to 4

Pot Roast

INGREDIENTS:

    2 large onions
    1 large carrot
    2 sweet peppers
    3-pound roast (beef or pork)
    3 cups water
    Salt and pepper to taste

1. Slice onions, carrot, and peppers.
2. Put vegetables, water, seasonings, and roast in a Crock-Pot.
3. Cook overnight at lowest setting (or until meat falls away from bone).
4. If you don't have a Crock-Pot, heat oven to 325 degrees and cook in a Dutch oven (large pot or pan) for approximately 2 to 3 hours.

Serves 8 to 12 depending on size of roast

Cornish Game Hen

One of Ray's favorites.

INGREDIENTS:

    1 whole hen with giblets
    4 stalks celery

1 cup sliced fresh mushrooms
¼ cup real bacon (uncured) bits
½ onion
1 teaspoon poultry seasoning
4 tablespoons bacon (uncured) grease

1. Preheat oven to 350 degrees.
2. Wash hen and stuff with seasoned, chopped giblets and vegetables.
3. Smear seasoned bacon grease on outside of hen and place in roasting pan.
4. Bake for 20 minutes per pound of hen plus 20 minutes for stuffing (which, when done, should be a golden brown color), basting every 30 minutes.

Serves 2 to 4

Baked Chicken with Herbs

INGREDIENTS:
    One 3- to 4-pound chicken
    2 tablespoons olive oil
    Salt and pepper to taste (both optional)
    2 to 3 teaspoons dried herbs of your choice (rosemary, thyme, tarragon, sage, etc.)

1. Preheat oven to 350 degrees.
2. Wash chicken and pat dry with paper towels.
3. Rub skin of chicken with olive oil. (If using salt or pepper or both, coat chicken evenly with them now.)
4. To bring out the flavor of the dried herbs (use only one at a time), rub vigorously back and forth in palms or crush in a mortar.
5. Rub entire surface of chicken with herbs.

6. Place in baking dish large enough to hold, breast side up.

7. Bake for approximately 1½ hours total. After first half hour check for juices in pan. Once juices appear, baste chicken about every 15 to 20 minutes until done. Chicken is done when meat thermometer placed in the thickest part of the meat (not touching a bone) reads 185 degrees, or when leg joint doesn't wiggle and juices from pierced leg-thigh joint are clear (the best way to learn how to tell when a chicken is done is to cook a few and learn). If you doubt your ability, investing in a $3.00 meat thermometer will save you much time and guessing.

VARIATION: If you want to give the chicken more flavor, mix the juice of one lemon with the olive oil, and put the two halves of the lemon rind in the chicken's cavity during the baking (remove rind before serving).

Serves 4 to 6

Lemon Thyme Pesto Chicken

INGREDIENTS:

> 2 tablespoons dried thyme (or, if available, 6 tablespoons fresh)
> Juice of ½ small lemon
> 2 to 3 tablespoons extra virgin olive oil
> Salt and freshly ground black pepper to taste
> 1 clove garlic, minced
> One 3- to 4-pound chicken

1. Preheat oven to 350 degrees.

2. Combine all ingredients (except chicken) and mix thoroughly. (The best way is to grind them with a mortar and pestle,

but if you don't have one, put everything in a small bowl and stir vigorously so as to release the essential oils from the thyme and garlic.)

3. Coat chicken with mixture and bake for approximately 1½ to 2 hours. After the first hour the chicken should begin to release its juices. Baste the chicken with the juices every 15 to 20 minutes until done.

Serves 4 to 6

NOTE: If you have already prepared Pesto (page 136), you can coat the chicken with it and cook the chicken in the manner described above in step 3.

Spicy Pork Chops

INGREDIENTS:
 4 tablespoons bacon grease (or 5 tablespoons olive oil)
 4 pork chops (thick)
 1 large onion
 2 cloves garlic
 1 teaspoon ground cumin
 1 teaspoon oregano
 1½ teaspoons salt (2 teaspoons salt if using olive oil)
 2 tablespoons chili powder
 1 cup tomato sauce

1. Put grease (or oil) in a large, deep skillet over medium heat.
2. When grease is hot (sizzling), put pork chops in pan and allow to brown fully.
3. Put onion and garlic in pan, and sauté until soft.

4. Add herbs, seasonings (only 1 tablespoon chili powder), and tomato paste. Cover skillet, lower heat, and allow to simmer for 8 to 10 minutes.

5. Uncover, add second tablespoon chili powder, and flip chops. Simmer until chops are tender.

6. Serve hot.

7. Optional: Garnish plate with sides of guacamole and salsa (see recipes).

Serves 2 to 4

Snacks

Jerky

Jerked meat makes a convenient snack food for road trips or carrying to the office, and it is quite simple to make.

INGREDIENTS:

As much lean red meat (beef, venison) as you want

Classically, jerky is made by removing all fat from the meat, cutting meat into ¼-inch strips, and laying the strips out to dry in the sun for 1 to 2 days. If you elect to use an oven, heat (do not cook) the strips at a very low temperature (90 to 100 degrees) until they are thoroughly dried. (A food dehydrator is preferable.) As NeanderThin jerky is not sugar-cured and contains no preservatives, it may become moldy in a warm, humid environment. If you want to keep it for an extended period of time (more than a week), store it in your freezer.

6 pounds raw meat yields 1 pound jerky

Pemmican

Pemmican was relied on heavily by native North Americans when traveling. A high-energy food that keeps for an extended period of time without refrigeration (hundreds of years if stored properly), pemmican also makes a great snack for the modern hunter-gatherer.

INGREDIENTS:

1 pound suet (beef fat)
1 pound dried Jerky (page 146)

1. Render (melt) the suet in a pan (preferably cast-iron). The purpose of rendering the fat is to remove all the water contained in it. Use enough heat to bring the melted suet to a slow bubbling. Allow it to cool and repeat the process. (Placing a pan of suet in a pre-heated oven heated to 250 degrees for approximately 2 hours will also remove all the water content.) Remove any solids from the final product by straining the liquid fat. If the suet smokes when being melted, turn down the heat. There is a danger of fire if the suet is allowed to smoke too long.

2. Pound jerky into a fine powder (a food processor can make this process much easier) and add to the rendered suet.

3. While the mixture is still liquid, pour into muffin pan. When the fat hardens, you will have solid cakes.

Serves 8 to 12 (a little bit goes a long way)

TIPS: Wrap individual cakes in wax paper for convenience, as pemmican is greasy.

Dried berries can be added to the recipe during cooking, if it suits your taste.

Frozen Banana

A banana contains a lot of carbohydrates. If you are trying to lose weight, its best to avoid foods high in carbohydrates. Eating a frozen banana once in a while won't impede your efforts if you're simply trying to maintain your current weight. Just don't overindulge.

INGREDIENTS:

1 banana
1 metal or wooden skewer
Almond butter
Shredded coconut

1. Peel banana. Insert skewer into banana lengthwise.
2. Spread nut butter over entire banana.
3. Roll in coconut.
4. Place on wax paper.
5. Freeze for 2 hours.

Serves 1

NeanderThin Cookies

Great for kids.

INGREDIENTS:

1 cup almond butter
1 whole large egg
2 tablespoons unsweetened applesauce
½ cup raisins
1 tablespoon coconut oil

1. Preheat oven to 375 degrees.
2. Mix ingredients into thick batter (not a dough).
3. Drop batter by tablespoons onto a cookie sheet greased with coconut oil.
4. Bake until golden brown (about 10 to 12 minutes). Check cookies occasionally to ensure they don't burn.
5. Serve warm.

Serves 4 to 6

Coconut Ice Cream

INGREDIENTS:

1 ripe coconut (thick, white flesh)
2 pints canned coconut milk

1. Crack coconut using a hammer and a screwdriver to extract the milk.
2. Scoop out the flesh and put about ½ pound of flesh and 2 pints of canned coconut milk in a blender. Blend at moderate speed.
3. Pour extracted milk into blender and add fruit (blueberries, raspberries, peaches, etc.) if desired. Blend at same speed.
4. Put the mixture into a bowl and place in freezer. Stir frequently.
5. When mixture is cold and thick (hard to stir), it's ready to eat.

Serves 2 to 3

Apple Pie

Apple pie shouldn't be a regular part of your diet. This recipe has a considerable amount of sugar per serving, so it should only be eaten as a treat. If you like a thicker crust, add more pecan flour. Experiment with crust ingredients if you like. Try adding a raw egg or a teaspoon of honey.

CRUST INGREDIENTS:
⅔ cup pecan flour
4 large dates
¼ cup applesauce (see recipe or use store-bought variety without preservatives)
1 tablespoon water

FILLING INGREDIENTS:
1 or 2 apples, chopped
¼ teaspoon cinnamon
⅛ teaspoon nutmeg
½ teaspoon lemon juice (optional)

1. Use a blender or an electric mixer to blend the crust ingredients.
2. Add filling ingredients in a bowl, mix together, and spread evenly over crust.
3. Place pie in oven at 350 degrees for 3 to 5 minutes.
4. Serve hot.

Serves 5 to 8

MENU SUGGESTIONS

This section contains meal suggestions for breakfast, lunch, dinner, and snacks. The list of snacks is separated into categories of low, moderate, and high-carbohydrate snacks. Stick mostly to snacks from the low-carb list to avoid eating too many carbohydrates. Eat moderate and high-carb snacks only occasionally—especially if you need to lose body fat or have a problem with high blood cholesterol or insulin levels.

Breakfast

2 large pork chops, fried
2 eggs
¼ slice cantaloupe

5 Deviled Eggs (page 121)
4 homemade sausage patties
1 glass freshly squeezed grapefruit juice

8 strips bacon (uncured, low sodium)
3 eggs
One 8-ounce glass freshly squeezed grapefruit juice

12-ounce rib eye steak (rare)
1 sliced pear

Omelet (3 eggs, bacon, onion, green pepper, tomato)
One 8-ounce glass freshly squeezed orange juice

6 venison sausage patties (homemade, low sodium)
Vegetable juice (low sodium)

½ pound Pemmican (page 147)
1 bowl strawberries, blueberries, and fresh coconut
1 cup fresh almond milk poured over berries and coconut
1 cup peppermint tea

4 pork spareribs (leftovers)
Eggs scrambled with mushroom, onion, and green peppers
Salsa (page 135) topping for scrambled eggs
1 cup Earl Grey tea

1 bowl (or more) Chicken Soup (page 119) (leftover, on a cold winter day)
1 cup hot cider

4 apple quarters dipped in almond butter
¼ pound Pemmican (page 147)
1 glass freshly squeezed citrus juice (tangerine, orange, grapefruit)

2 pork chops, broiled
1 bowl Applesauce (page 114) (spread on pork chops)
1 cup green tea

Lunch and Dinner

Chili (page 117)
Tossed salad with A Vinegarless Vinaigrette (page 131)
Cucumber slices
Iced tea

Ground beef with pasta sauce
Steamed broccoli and cauliflower
½ cup almonds
½ cup water with lemon

Barbecued pork spareribs (NeanderThin Barbecue Sauce [page 135])
Side of sliced onions

NeanderThin Slaw (see page 130)
1 glass mineral water (flavored with freshly squeezed orange juice)

One 16-ounce prime rib (rare)
Wild green salad (with NeanderThin Mayonnaise dressing [page 132])
Sweet pepper and tomato slices
Hot tea

Pot Roast (page 142)
Tossed salad with A Vinegarless Vinaigrette (page 131)
Steamed cauliflower and yellow squash
1 glass iced tea

1½ pounds boiled shrimp
Tossed salad (liberal amounts of avocado oil and lemon juice for dressing)
1 cup filberts
1 glass iced herbal tea

2 baked chicken leg quarters (marinade: lemon juice, rosemary, oregano, thyme)
Sliced veggies (celery, sweet pepper, carrots)
Low-carb fruit salad (pears, oranges, strawberries, and honeydew melon)
1 glass Perrier mineral water

3 Spicy Pork Chops (page 145)
Green tomatillo sauce (bought at health food store)
NeanderThin Guacamole (page 128)
Tossed salad (romaine lettuce, escarole, cabbage, kale, parsley, garlic, cucumber, carrots)

1 sliced peach
1 glass iced tea

Lemon Thyme Pesto Chicken (page 144)
Venetian Salad (page 129)
Sliced veggies with Pesto (page 136)
1 glass water

2 bowls Green Chili Stew (page 118)
Sliced veggies (broccoli, cauliflower, celery, radishes)
1 cup nut mix (filberts, hazelnuts, walnuts)
1 cup hot tea

2 bowls Chicken Soup (page 119)
Steamed asparagus
1 small bowl Waldorf Salad (page 126)
1 glass water

2 hamburger patties (with Mom's Ketchup [page 133] and NeanderThin Mayonnaise [page 132])
2 large lettuce leaves
½ avocado, sliced
1 tomato slice
2 onion slices
1 glass Perrier mineral water (flavored with freshly squeezed orange juice)

2 large bowls Tuna Salad with Onion, Avocado, and Egg (page 127)
1 glass iced tea

½ rotisserie chicken (from deli)
1 cup Roman Egg Drop Soup (page 120)
2 cups peppermint tea

3 Shish Kebabs (page 138)
1 cup cooked spinach
1 plum
1 glass Nut Milk (page 114)

5 barbecued chicken drumsticks
Slaw (page 130)
1 glass iced tea

Snacks

Low Carbohydrate

Pork rinds (low sodium) and almond butter
Pork rinds (low sodium) and salsa
Oysters on the half-shell with lemon (at oyster bar)
Boiled shrimp
Nuts (walnuts, chestnuts, pecans, Brazil nuts, hazelnuts)
Pemmican (page 147)
Jerky (page 146)
NeanderThin Guacamole (page 128) and sliced veggies (celery, sweet pepper, broccoli, cauliflower)
Trail mix (assorted nuts and a small amount of dried fruit for taste)
Vegetable slices dipped in NeanderThin Mayonnaise (page 132)
Sardines (packed in olive oil, water, or tomato sauce)
Leftover barbecued ribs
Fresh vegetable juice (made in juicer; celery, sweet pepper, broccoli, spinach, cucumber, parsley, 1 small carrot, and several tomatoes; lots of pulp; add cayenne pepper for spice; add 1 or 2 tablespoons flaxseed oil for essential fatty acid supplement)

Additional Low-Carbohydrate Snacks
Boiled eggs
Deviled Eggs (page 121)
A few strips of bacon (uncured, low sodium)
Handful of sliced dried coconut
3 eggs scrambled
Leftover Chili (page 117)
Leftover Chicken Soup (page 119)
Leftover Green Chili Stew (page 118)
Can of tuna fish (boring but easy; pour on some olive oil or A Vinegarless Vinaigrette [page 131] for extra fat and flavor)

Moderate Carbohydrate
Frozen fruit slush (ice, berries, freshly squeezed orange juice)
Low-sugar fruit salad (peaches, pears, berries, nectarines, orange, melon balls)
Coconut Ice Cream (page 149)
Freshly squeezed juice (apple, orange, etc.) frozen in popsicle trays

High Carbohydrate (for special occasions;
not for daily snacking)
Waldorf Salad (page 126)
Apple Pie (page 149)
Frozen Banana (page 148)
Fruit smoothie (banana, water, assorted fruit, and fruit juice)
Dried fruit

A ONE-WEEK FOOD DIARY

The following sample food diary shows what I might eat during the week. It doesn't include liquid intake. Throughout a normal day I drink approximately 2 to 4 liters of purified water and tea (green and black). If I go out of the house, I carry a bottle of water or a thermos of tea. I don't eat out very often because I prefer to cook my own food. I work at home, and meals at home are less expensive.

Monday

Breakfast
Omelet (3 eggs*) cooked in olive oil at low heat
6 strips uncured bacon†(fried in a second pan)
small glass freshly squeezed orange juice

Snack
½ cup walnuts
1 strip Jerky (page 146)
1 small plum

Lunch
¾ pound grilled salmon
½ cup Brazil nuts
4 cups tossed salad (kale, romaine lettuce, chard, dill, parsley)
with 4 tablespoons A Vinegarless Vinaigrette (page 131) and
1 tablespoon flaxseed oil

Snack
1 tin sardines (packed in olive oil)

---

* I use eggs enriched with omega-3 fatty acids.
† I soak my bacon overnight in a cold pan of water in the refrigerator. Soaking removes the sugar and salt content of the bacon, as sugar and salt are water soluble.

Dinner

½ pound sliced beef (eye of round)

Tossed salad (left over from lunch) with 4 tablespoons A Vinegarless Vinaigrette (page 131)

1 medium-size apple

Snack

1 strip Jerky (page 146)

2 cups mixed nuts (Brazil nuts, walnuts, almonds)

Tuesday

Breakfast

4 eggs scrambled with chopped broccoli, onions, tomatoes, and garlic; cooked in olive oil on low heat

6 strips uncured bacon (fried in a second pan)

1 small glass unfiltered apple juice (from health food store)

Snack

½ cup almonds

1 strip Jerky (page 146)

Lunch

2 medium-size chicken breasts (marinated in NeanderThin Barbecue Sauce [page 135])

1 large avocado (sliced)

Tossed salad (green leaf lettuce, green onions, garlic, A Vinegarless Vinaigrette [page 131])

1 cup strawberries

Snack

1 tin sardines (packed in olive oil)

1 medium-size tomato (sliced)

Dinner
> ¾ pound tuna salad (canned tuna packed in spring water,
> NeanderThin Mayonnaise [page 132], chopped celery)
> 3 cups steamed broccoli

Snack
> ½ cup Pemmican (page 147)
> 1 cup mixed nuts (macadamia nuts, Brazil nuts, walnuts)

Wednesday

Breakfast
> 12-ounce steak with 2 eggs
> Small glass orange juice
> Hot tea with lemon

Lunch
> Double meat hamburger (with lettuce, tomato, and onion—
> throw away the bun)
> Medium iced tea

Snack
> 1 bottle mineral water
> 1 apple
> 1 small bag of almonds

Dinner
> 6 medium-size shrimp (boiled, not fried)
> 6 raw oysters with lemon
> 12-ounce grilled tuna steak
> Dinner salad
> Iced tea

Snack
1 cup Brazil nuts
½ cup Pemmican (page 147)

Thursday

Breakfast
½ grapefruit
1 large bowl Roman Egg Drop Soup (page 120)

Snack
½ cup macadamia nuts
1 sliced kiwi

Lunch
½ cup almonds
4 cups Simple, Perfect Chicken Salad (page 127) plus 1 table-spoon flaxseed oil served on a bed of lettuce

Snack
1 large avocado
1 slice Jerky (page 146)

Dinner
¼ cantaloupe
1 pound grilled halibut
Tossed salad with 4 tablespoons A Vinegarless Vinaigrette (page 131)

Snack
½ cup Pemmican (page 147)

Friday
Breakfast
Shrimp omelet
1 Valencia orange

Snack
1 tin sardines (packed in olive oil)

Lunch
2 Cold Shrimp-Stuffed Avocados (page 122)
3 cups steamed broccoli
1 small nectarine

Snack
1½ cups nut mix (hazelnuts, walnuts)
1 slice Jerky (page 146)

Dinner
2 bowls Chili (page 117)
2 cups Waldorf Salad (page 126)

Snack
1 cup leftover Chili
1 cup leftover Waldorf Salad

Saturday
Breakfast
1 small glass unfiltered pear juice (from health food store)
2 pork tenderloin steaks
2 scrambled eggs

Snack
1 cup Pemmican (page 147)

Lunch
1 small rabbit (cooked over an open fire)
3 fish oil capsules (1,000 milligrams)

Snack
3 handfuls nut mix
½ cup Pemmican (page 147)

Dinner
2 Grilled Venison Steaks (page 137)
Wild green salad
2 cups steamed cauliflower
1 bowl Applesauce (page 114)

Sunday
Breakfast
3 scrambled eggs cooked in olive oil
1 cup NeanderThin Guacamole (page 128)
1 cup Salsa (page 135)

Lunch
½ pound baked fish with lemon juice
Tossed salad
2 Deviled Eggs (page 121)
Small bowl strawberries
Iced tea

Snack
½ cup Pemmican (page 147)
3 cups mixed nuts (macadamia nuts, walnuts, almonds, Brazil nuts)
1 liter carbonated water (flavored with orange juice)

Dinner
    1 bowl leftover Chili
    1 cup leftover Waldorf Salad
    2 cups leftover wild field green salad (3 tablespoons A Vinegar-less Vinaigrette [page 131], 1 tablespoon flaxseed oil)

CHAPTER THIRTEEN

Frequently Asked Questions

Q: Should I consult my physician before starting the NeanderThin diet?

A: Yes. Before embarking on any dietary program, you should consult your physician. It will not hurt to get a good summary of your current health status in order to chart any improvements. As your body cannot *require* anything that, in nature, it cannot *acquire,* your doctor should have no problem with your adopting the NeanderThin program.

Q: Don't the high levels of red meat and animal fat in the NeanderThin program lead to cardiovascular disease?

A: Approximately half the fat in red meat consists of stearic acid, a powerful antioxidant, that reduces your risk of both arteriosclerosis and cancer. Remember that heart disease is an immune system problem caused by the ingestion of alien proteins, not saturated fat. High cholesterol is typically the body's response to high blood insulin and glucose levels resulting from a high-carbohydrate diet. Practicing NeanderThin has been shown to lower blood insulin and glucose levels resulting in improved blood cholesterol ratios (LDL/HDL and total cholesterol/HDL).

The three most effective methods of elevating your blood cholesterol level are as follows (in order of decreasing risk):

1. Drinking coffee that has not been percolated or filtered through paper (see Urgert in Bibliography);
2. Eating a low-fat, high-carbohydrate diet (24 percent increase in LDL-cholesterol in 6 weeks; see Garg in Bibliography);
3. Eating vegetable oils thickened by hydrogenation (aka trans-fatty acids; there is a much stronger correlation—two times greater—between high LDL levels and trans-fatty acids than between LDL and saturated fat; see Ascherio and Willet in Bibliography).

Obviously, excessive blood cholesterol is undesirable, and these three practices are highly inadvisable.

Trying to reduce fat consumption while following the principles of the NeanderThin program will only reduce metabolism, produce fatigue, and slow weight loss. As stated above, low-fat diets have been shown to dramatically increase LDL ("bad") cholesterol and lipid levels in some individuals (see Garg in Bibliography). Remember that eating saturated fat from natural sources isn't unsafe—it's the body's defensive response to alien proteins in unnatural foods that leads to autoimmune disease (such as heart disease).

Consider the following quote from a paper on vegetarianism written by researcher H. Leon Abrams:

> . . . [M]illions of Americans are convinced that by not eating meat, eggs, and dairy products and by consuming only plant fats (polyunsaturated fats) they will greatly reduce their chances of suffering from heart disease that afflicts and kills a million or more Americans every year. Scrutinization of the facts shows that they have been lulled into a false sense of security. They fail to know or understand the following facts that are never carried in [related] advertisements:

1. There is no positive or direct scientific proof that eating foods high in cholesterol raises serum cholesterol levels.
2. There is no positive or direct proof that high cholesterol levels result in heart disease.
3. There is no positive or direct proof that lowering cholesterol levels will reduce one's susceptibility to heart disease.
4. Consuming great quantities of polyunsaturated fats or oils may be detrimental to health.

In an article titled "The Three Weak Links in the Diet-Heart Disease Connection" published in *Nutrition Today* (see Bibliography), Dr. Raymond Reiser shows as erroneous the popular notion that high blood cholesterol levels are linked with a diet high in animal fat and cholesterol content. He demonstrates the following:

1. Not all persons are equally at risk for coronary disease when consuming diets high in animal fat and cholesterol.

2. Risk for heart disease does not necessarily increase as serum cholesterol levels increase.

3. Blood cholesterol levels cannot be controlled by removing foods from the diet that are rich in animal fat and cholesterol.

Finally, and perhaps most authoritatively, Dr. Michael De Bakey, the world-famous cardiac surgeon, has shown that only 30 to 40 percent of people with heart disease have elevated serum cholesterol levels. Dr. De Bakey found no definite connection between atherosclerotic disease and high blood cholesterol (see De Bakey and Abrams in Bibliography).

Q: I'm not overweight. Why should I eat this way?
A: Most people who adopt NeanderThin are not overweight (at least for very long). Even a person of average weight will experience dramatic improvements in his overall health, energy level,

and fitness within a few weeks of adopting the NeanderThin program.

Even if you are not presently overweight, your genetics may betray you 20 years from now. By eating like a hunter-gatherer you greatly reduce your risk of succumbing to autoimmune disease (95 percent of Americans die of autoimmune-related diseases).

You will not become too thin eating this way. Once you have reached your optimal body composition, you will remain there as long as you follow the program.

The NeanderThin view also provides environmental, spiritual, and political benefits for many.

Q: To lose weight should I reduce my fat intake?

A: No. If you are trying to lose weight you are trying to metabolize your own body fats. As your own fat is animal fat, it is important to trigger this metabolic process by ingesting animal fat.

Q: As NeanderThin cuts out whole categories of food, should I take vitamin and mineral supplements?

A: Vitamins are enzymes used by the body to metabolize food. When you eat unnatural foods they are used up faster than the body can replace them. This leads to vitamin deficiencies. By avoiding the forbidden fruits and eating a wide variety of natural foods, the need for vitamin and mineral supplements is eliminated.

Q: NeanderThin seems awfully strict. Aren't there easier ways to lose weight?

A: The only other way to lose weight involves caloric restriction and regular strenuous exercise. Like NeanderThin, this regimen must be continued for a lifetime to keep the weight off. The resulting hunger from starvation rations and the high risk of injury from strenuous exercise make this approach very difficult, if not impossible, for most who try it. With NeanderThin the cravings for forbidden fruits diminish with time, but with caloric restriction you will often be hungry and unable to eat your fill. The optional "NeanderFit" exercise program is designed to develop muscle rather than burn calories. So it is not nearly as strenuous and time-consuming as programs focusing primarily on weight loss. Of course, by adding muscle you increase your metabolism and speed the process of losing undesired body fat. As NeanderFit is a moderate exercise program, you will reduce the risk of injury associated with more strenuous exercise programs.

Q: I find it difficult to stick to the NeanderThin diet 100 percent. Will a modified version of the plan work for me?

A: The extent to which you can partake of the forbidden fruits can be determined only by experimenting with these foods after an extended period (several weeks at least) of being on the NeanderThin program exclusively. The least taboo of the forbidden fruits include dairy products (such as butter, yogurt, and cheese) and fruit-based alcohol (wine and champagne). While we highly recommend against the inclusion of any technology-dependent foods in your diet, as an individual you may find that including small amounts of dairy, fruit alcohol, and grains or grain-based products will produce no significant health problems. Low-carbohydrate diet programs recommended by several doctors—Atkins, Eades and Eades, Irwin Stillman, Simopoulos, Voegtlin, et al.—present less strict approaches to low-carbohydrate dieting, while adhering to the spirit of Paleo-lithic nutrition. If you find the NeanderThin program to be impractical in your circumstances, you might want to consider adopting one of these plans.

Having stated the above, it is important to reiterate that the NeanderThin program is based on the authors' research into the connection between autoimmune disease (including obesity) and agricultural foods. For those who adopt NeanderThin in hopes of alleviating the effects of autoimmune disorders, complete abstinence from the forbidden foods is highly recommended. It is impossible to determine the exact amount of alien protein exposure that any particular individual can sustain without contracting immune system problems. What one person can eat without negative results may cause severe symptoms in another even when eaten in small quantities. Regular consumption of technology-dependent foods is the dietary equivalent of Russian roulette.

Concerning practicality, the authors have followed NeanderThin for a combined total of 23 years (and over 100 years if you include Ray's six siblings). In our experience, strict adherence to NeanderThin is possible in almost any situation. There are plenty of acceptable food options available in most restaurants, and most restaurants will allow you to tailor menu items to fit dietary restrictions—after all, you're the customer, and they want your money. Also, there are many foods that you can carry conveniently when traveling (e.g., jerky, pemmican, nuts, trail mixes, fruit). With minimal creativity and dedication, almost anyone can eat this way for the rest of his life.

Q: My dog is overweight. Will NeanderThin work for him?

A: In nature, wolves and humans eat essentially the same foods. In fact, some scientists postulate this as the reason for wolves becoming the first domesticated animals. NeanderThin table scraps supplemented by raw meats (cheap cuts and organ) will provide the optimum diet for your dog and have him in good shape very soon. This diet is no more expensive than commercial dog foods.

Q: Can I still drink alcohol?

A: All alcohol is forbidden fruit and should be avoided. If you must drink, small amounts of wine are the least offensive choice within NeanderThin guidelines.

Q: Is NeanderThin safe during pregnancy?

A: As hunter-gatherers have the easiest births and the lowest incidence of birth defects, it is not only safe but is preferred. But before adopting any dietary changes, you must consult your family physician or obstetrician. The pregnant woman craves added nutrients to nourish and sustain herself and her developing baby. The mother's immune system is also working hard to protect mother and child, so care must be taken to avoid the forbidden fruits while satisfying cravings by increasing dietary diversity. In this way the nausea common in pregnancy can be greatly reduced if not eliminated.

Q: Since the inception of technology, hasn't the human body evolved to allow consumption of the forbidden fruits?

A: Humans have eaten technology-dependent foods for only 10,000 years or so. This amount of time equals approximately 300 generations. There are several breeds of chickens available with much longer pedigrees than humans. All of these breeds thrive on essentially the same blend of nutrients optimal for their jungle forebears.

Even small evolutionary changes take hundreds of thousands of years (some scientists say millions of years) to occur. For humans to adapt to foods that are not edible to any other primate would involve vast changes in our immune system as expressed in our DNA. For us to mutate to a form outside of the order *Primata* would be considered a huge evolutionary change. We are essentially the same creatures we were tens of thousands of years before the Neolithic Revolution.

Q: How long will it take me to lose weight following NeanderThin?

A: It depends upon how overweight you are and how long it took you to become that way. If you are very heavy, initial weight loss may be very dramatic (3 to 5 pounds per week). As you approach your ideal weight, this loss will slow and the last 10 or 20 pounds may take much longer (2 to 3 years). The process may be accelerated by lowering intake of high-carbohydrate foods (dried fruits, juices, nuts, etc.) and increasing moderate exercise (walking, golf, avoiding elevators, power parking, etc.). Adding muscle mass to your body through strength training will also increase your metabolism and speed weight loss.

Q: I'm an endurance athlete, and I usually load up on carbohydrates the day before an event. Since NeanderThin discourages high-carbohydrate intake, will I be able to perform at my peak while on the diet?

A: A recent study at the State University of New York at Buffalo debunks the theory behind "carbo-loading." Researchers discovered that endurance athletes performed better when on a high-fat, low-carbohydrate diet regimen than on their standard high-carbohydrate, low-fat diets.

The study was performed in three stages, increasing the percentage of fat during the second two stages, the third stage diet being the highest in fat (45 percent). Each stage lasted 4 weeks, allowing each athlete's body time to acclimate to the new percentage of fat in the diet. At the conclusion of each stage, each athlete performed a series of endurance tests. At the end of the 12-week test, the results indicated the following:

1. Overall endurance improved by 14 percent during the third stage diet composed of 45 percent fat.

2. Fatigue related to exercise decreased the most when the athletes ate the third stage, highest-fat diet.

3. The athletes most efficiently used stored body fat for energy when on the fattiest diet and metabolized fat the least efficiently on the first stage, the low-fat diet.

4. After adopting the higher fat diets, the athletes' immune

responses were heightened, resulting in increased white blood cell counts (immunological agents) and reduced counts of inflammatory agents.

Most significantly, it was discovered that the body takes weeks to acclimate to a diet higher in fat content than previously consumed. Studies that don't allow for an acclimation period will provide skewed results (see Raloff in Bibliography).

Q: I love animals. Can I practice NeanderThin as a vegetarian?

A: No. Without red meat the human body lacks the enzymes to process iron. Iron deficiency may be responsible for the high incidence of retardation, birth defects, and weakened physical condition endemic in vegetarian societies. Without the proteins contained in the forbidden fruits (grains, beans, dairy products), severe protein deficiencies will occur, which could be life threatening.

As the principle cause of animal extinction and death is the plow and not the slaughterhouse, vegetarians actually kill more animals through starvation and habitat destruction than does the meat-eater through his dietary habits. All the plants and animals that once inhabited the cultivated land must be killed to provide space for vegetable crops. Plowing accomplishes this "ecocide" very efficiently, but plowing also causes topsoil to erode by exposing it to wind and rain. Erosion can cause even the most fertile fields to become barren, sometimes in less than 100 years of cultivation. Some life-forms that inhibit good crop yields survive the onslaught of the plow. Such organisms (insects, weeds, etc.) must be fought using herbicides and insecticides. The more dependent a population is on vegetable crops, the more wild animal and plant habitats it must destroy to feed itself. Meat production is usually less damaging to plant and animal habitats—especially when the animals are range fed. In fact, it is for this reason that the person wearing a fur coat has killed fewer than 10 percent of the animals killed by the person wearing a cotton coat (cotton is one of the most ecologically damaging crops grown today, second only, perhaps, to rice). Perhaps the only species that are not endangered in our modern world are domestic animals. Any knowledgeable primatologist will tell you that there are no vegetarian primates. Remember that predation is a part of nature. Humans are designed by nature to be predators. A vegetarian diet is no more natural for a human than a diet of Cheerios would be for a lion. And humans kill animals much more quickly and compassionately than lions or any other predator. We have a responsibility to treat our domestic animals with compassion and respect. However, we cannot do this by removing ourselves from our rightful place in the planetary food chain.

Q: Once I have reached my weight goal, can I return to normal foods?

A: No. Any weight lost will be regained even more quickly than it was originally lost. It cannot be overemphasized that it is not the calories or fat content that produces the weight gain, as has been traditionally proposed; instead, it is the alien proteins present in the forbidden fruits that cause an overweight condition.

Q: According to your theory, shouldn't I eat all my food raw?

A: In a perfect world, yes. But modern farming and food processing techniques preclude this practice. Meats, poultry, eggs, and seafood are prone to contamination by bacteria (salmonella, e. coli, etc.) and parasites (trichinosis, tapeworms, etc.) and should be cooked or dried at least enough to sterilize them. When available, irradiated foods will eliminate this risk and make steak tartar and raw eggs much more possible. Fruit and vegetables in the diet can compensate for the slight loss of vitamins and nutrients caused by light cooking, but these should be washed thoroughly to remove bacteria, germs, and pesticide residue.

Q: Are prepackaged convenience foods (frozen, canned, microwavable, etc.) allowed in the NeanderThin program?

A: Although not categorically eliminated, most prepackaged foods contain one or more of the forbidden fruits and should be avoided. On a case-by-case basis, this can be determined only by carefully reading labels. Because of their low government subsidy costs, unnatural foods are often used as cheap fillers in a wide variety of products. Often, soy is added to meat products, flavored corn syrup is substituted in fruit juices, and starch from corn is added to almost anything.

Some prepackaged foods such as frozen fruit juices are lacking for what is not there. Fruit juice from concentrate has had most of the fiber, protein, and vitamins removed, leaving only the sugar, and should, therefore, not be seen as a substitute for real fruit juice or fresh fruit.

Q: I have food allergies. Will this diet work for me?

A: As the most common food allergies are reactions to corn, wheat, and milk, the NeanderThin program should be excellent for individuals suffering from conditions caused by their consumption. Less common are allergic reactions to seafood. As these were among the last foodstuffs added to the human diet before the Neolithic Revolution, it is not surprising that some humans cannot tolerate seafood. Should you have these allergic reactions, you must continue to avoid seafood.

Individuals who experience allergies to other foods such as eggs, certain nuts, and fruits should continue to avoid these foods. Fear not, however, as, regardless of the severity of the food allergy, acceptable substitutes can always be found and the NeanderThin program continued.

Q: Won't my friends think that I'm weird if I eat this way?

A: At first, yes, as you are going against thousands of years of cultural programming; but as your condition improves, any disdain will be replaced by curiosity. As your attitude becomes more positive, you will also become more prone to zealotry, which others may find obnoxious. Try to avoid this by not criticizing everything they eat. Instead, lead by example.

Q: Isn't NeanderThin expensive?
A: It may seem so at first. For the price of a pound of meat, you can buy a bushel of government-subsidized wheat. But by eating out less and avoiding unnecessary medical costs associated with the forbidden fruits, the hunter-gatherer comes out ahead. Remember that slim people often get more raises and make more money, and people with disabilities caused by immune system diseases often find it hard to work at all. There is no better investment than your own body.

Q: Shouldn't I exercise more?
A: Yes, but only in moderation. Strenuous exercise has more risks than benefits and should be avoided. The best exercise is walking, bearing in mind that it is the time spent and not the distance covered that counts. Any activity pursued with this rule of thumb in mind—such as walking your dog, bird watching, falconry, golf, etc.—is excellent. More intense forms of exercise should be added in moderation when your fitness level has improved. As you lose weight your joints will be stressed much less by sudden movements. As your muscle tone improves, the potential for muscle strain will also be reduced.

Mental activity is also a form of exercise. Try to use your increased energy to improve and not just entertain—i.e., distract—your mind. You will improve not only your physical health but may also improve your intellectual abilities and overall outlook on life.

Q: Is NeanderThin good for children?
A: As many childhood conditions such as obesity, hyperactivity,

ear infections, frequent colds, juvenile diabetes, juvenile epilepsy, rickets, myopia, etc., have been shown to be diet related, the NeanderThin program is excellent for children. For the same reasons, breast-feeding is also highly recommended. Again, consult your pediatrician before making any dietary changes or embarking on any new nutritional program.

Children are often tempted by such goodies as milk and cookies served by well-meaning day care workers, teachers, or friends' parents. They must be educated from a very early age to avoid the forbidden foods.

Q: Why have I not heard of this before?

A: Quite simply, it is a matter of perspective. As modern humans, we tend to view all things through the lens of civilization. Our worldview is framed by a set of social and cultural parameters of which we are largely unaware and which distort our understanding of our biological and evolutionary origins.

What we call civilization is a continuous process, the origins of which lie in agrarian agricultural intensification. Cultures founded upon agrarian agricultural intensification began in several parts of the world, including the Fertile Crescent of the Middle East, the Indus River Valley of India, the Yellow River Valley of China, and the high plateaus of Peru.

Just as the Roman Empire was built for the production and distribution of bread and wine, so all civilizations promote activities that benefit the crop species that spawn them. Anthropologists often use the peculiarities of the life cycles of different crops to explain the differences found between cultures.

Agricultural plant species promote themselves through custom, religion, politics, manners, morals, and ethics. Since Gutenberg they have also used the mass media. Indeed a large part of all advertising is paid for by the forbidden fruits.

Just as the English House of Lords favored the large agrarian landholder, so the Great Compromise of 1787 ensured that the U.S. Senate gives greater representation to farmers than to urban tenants and building owners. This unequal balance of power only increases as the number of farmers becomes smaller in relationship to city populations (farmers presently make up approximately 1 percent of the U.S. population).

Also, the government promotes a food pyramid, favoring the forbidden fruits, which was brought about by the same sort of political forces that built the original pyramids.

All of the aforementioned forces have served to overwhelm the quiet voice of NeanderThin Man, leaving his views underrepresented in ethnic and anthropological studies. The chief reason, however, that you might not have heard of the Paleolithic diet before may simply be that in our modern, high-tech world, the simplest ideas and solutions often lie hidden in plain sight.

It is only since civilization has begun to face worldwide ecological disaster, caused by agricultural intensification, that the hunter-gatherer viewpoint has come to light, finding its voice in both the Deep Ecology movement and the new science of Paleolithic nutrition.

Q: Is NeanderThin good for the environment?

A: Since ancient times, the most destructive factor in the degradation of the environment has been monoculture agriculture. The production of wheat in ancient Sumeria transformed once-fertile plains into salt flats that remain sterile 5,000 years later. As well as depleting both the soil and water sources, monoculture agriculture also produces environmental damage by altering the delicate balance of natural ecosystems. World rice production in 1993, for instance, caused 155 million cases of malaria by providing breeding grounds for mosquitoes in the paddies. Human contact with ducks in the same rice paddies resulted in 500 million cases of influenza during the same year.

A frequently argued assertion is that our continued reliance on animal foods constitutes a highly inefficient use of scarce food resources. It is argued that domestic animals compete with humans for food, eating perhaps three times as much food as they provide for humans. This argument is based on the fallacy that the land used to raise domestic animals could be turned to use in raising plants. In fact, only 35 percent of Earth's landmass can be used for food production. The remaining landmass consists of mountains, deserts, cities, snow, ice, marshes, and other kinds of geographical features that render it useless for agricultural purposes.

Of the 35 percent of the world's usable land, only one third is suitable for growing crops. This portion of the 35 percent is predicted to shrink as a result of global warming caused by the greenhouse effect and the erosion inherently caused by agrarian agricultural practices.

The nature of the remaining two thirds of the usable land will only support the growth of plants that can be consumed by ruminant animals—not by humans. Only by raising domestic animals on this land can we derive any food value from the resources it offers. If we eliminated animal husbandry from our agricultural practices, two thirds of the world's land currently used for agriculture would become useless. The result would be a net loss in overall food production. (Source: Department of Animal Science at Oklahoma State University, web site at www.ansi.okstate.edu/breeds.)

Many environmentalists now believe the only way to preserve the environment is to return to our natural place on the food chain. Over time nature produces more nutrients per acre than any method of agriculture. Learning to intelligently harvest this natural bounty without destroying it is the biggest challenge facing modern man.

APPENDIX A

A Prehistoric Timeline

Phases of the Paleolithic	Human Genera & Species	Phases of the Pleistocene	Years Before Present
Upper Paleolithic			10,000 20,000 30,000 40,000
		Late Pleistocene	
	Homo sapiens		100,000
		Middle Pleistocene	200,000
			400,000 700,000
		Early Pleistocene	
	Homo erectus		1,000,000
Lower Paleolithic	*Homo babilis*		2,000,000
	Austra-lopithecus	Pliocene	5,000,000

APPENDIX B

Paleolithic Man and His Lifestyle

The emergence of hominids (savanna apes) in Africa preceded the first appearance of modern humans (genus *Homo*) by several million years. *Homo erectus,* considered to be the second of these proto-humans (preceded by *Homo habilis*), appeared approximately 1 million years ago during the early part of the Pleistocene Era (see Appendix A). *Homo erectus* was the first hominid to migrate north from the African continent.

Thus, modern humans can be seen as a creature of the Pleistocene. This geological epoch was characterized by rapid changes in the climate that began less dramatically several million years before. These climactic changes began when the rapid rise of the Himalaya mountains changed the earth's weather patterns and drastically lowered carbon dioxide (CO_2) levels in our atmosphere. Decreased CO_2 levels caused lower temperatures around the world. The reduction in CO_2 levels also favored the growth of grasses over plants with woody stems, such as trees and shrubs. These latter plants have less surface area devoted to photosynthesis and thrive in higher CO_2 conditions.

A Prehistory Lesson

Ice Ages lasting more than 100,000 years occurred during the Pleistocene. They were punctuated by shorter periods (10,000 years or so) of warmer weather called interglacial periods. As the glacial ice sheets covered more land and locked water in their incredible mass, sea levels decreased, forming land bridges between continents. Precipitation levels increased during the periods of glaciation resulting in formerly dry tropical savannas becoming extremely lush. This new savanna could support much larger animals. Larger animals evolved to exploit this new lushness.

When the short, warm interglacial periods began, these new larger species were forced to migrate toward the poles to follow the precipitation that was a result of glaciers (because of an effect similar to the Great Lakes Effect seen in the American Midwest). This area of higher precipitation followed the edge of the ice mass and was very similar in conditions throughout the world, allowing these larger animals to migrate east and west as well as north and south. The areas where these animals had evolved during the Ice Age had become too dry to support their increased body weight.

Because of mass migration during the interglacial warmings, these new animals spread to every part of the globe, often far from where they had first evolved. Collectively, the new larger animals are known as the Pleistocene megafauna. They included mammoths, woolly rhinoceroses, several species of large camels, giant ground sloths, and others. The new hominids (*Homos*) can be thought of as "mega-men" as they rapidly increased in height and brain size.

These hominids also developed new tools and methods of hunting that enabled them to take large game consistently for the first time. Even the largest Pleistocene animals became available as food sources through opportunistic killing (mud bogs, cliff falls, etc.) and scavenging of kills by larger predators. Man followed his Pleistocene prey during their interglacial migrations into all the landmasses contiguous to his original African home. He found himself in temperate regions for the first time.

The lush grasslands bordering the glaciers are now known as the steppe-tundra. These types of grasslands no longer exist anywhere on Earth. They were characterized by a lack of trees and abundant growth of grasses. On the steppe-tundra, the growth of trees was prevented by permafrost, deep snows in winter, and the action of the abundant ruminant (herbivore) population inhabiting the region. Tree forests bordered the steppe-tundra. Warmer temperatures and elevated CO_2 levels during the short interglacial periods favored the growth of these forests. During these short periods, the growth of the forests caused a narrowing of the steppe-tundra.

Although this band of steppe-tundra was perhaps never more than a few hundred miles wide, it extended around the globe and covered a large total area. The population densities of large mammals in this lush region far exceeded similar populations on the dry savannas of Africa and North America (e.g., buffalo populations) in historic times.

As well as being larger than animals found in temperate climates today, the Pleistocene megafauna were adapted to long winters of deep snow, having evolved the ability to store large amounts of body fat. Their fat stores were used when deep snows made grazing very difficult and cold weather increased calorie and insulation requirements. Unlike animals inhabiting the nearby forests, the megafauna depended on grass for their sustenance. The woody stems of trees and shrubs not covered by snow in the forests could not make for quality grazing. And the large mass of these animals, which helped them survive on the grasslands, would have been a major hindrance in the deep forests, as they would have been extremely vulnerable to forest predators.

The megafauna would begin to store fat when their bodies detected high levels of carbohydrates in their diets in the late summer and fall when the grasses they ate contained seeds. Similarly, humans began to develop a greater sensitivity to carbohydrates in the diet during the short season when edible fruits were available.

Although other apes also respond to high-carbohydrate foods in a similar manner, the tropical region where these apes are found exhibits a longer fruiting season, meaning that other apes did not develop a reliance on stored body fat for significant periods of time. The human ability to store body fat in response to increased carbohydrate consumption was not a necessary survival adaption required of apes in tropical climates.

During the winter, plant food was almost completely unavailable to humans in the steppe-tundra, so they adapted to eating only the meat, organs, and storage fat of ruminant (grass-eating) animals during this season. Winter conditions increased man's ability to take large animals, whose movement was restricted by deep snow. Cold conditions also made preserving meat possible by freezing, allowing humans to use much more meat from each kill.

Studies of contemporary Inuit (Eskimo) have shown that when people eat a totally carnivorous diet they must obtain at least 70 percent of their calories from fat, or they will face malnutrition (called "rabbit starvation" by the Inuit). When eating a diet so high in fat even for a short time, the human body is also better able to use its stored fat more efficiently. So when extreme Pleistocene winter conditions made hunting impossible or made game scarce, man could use the fat he stored during the summer and fall carbohydrate bingeing.

At the end of the last interglacial period—which began approximately 127,000 years ago—the forests and dry savannas covered most of the temperate and tropical world inhabited by humans. The little steppe-tundra that survived was confined to areas near the modern Arctic and Antarctic regions. As this most recent Ice Age began, it proceeded in fits and starts, punctuated by several periods that were much warmer than today's climate. It was only about 70,000 years ago that glaciation increased to the levels seen in the previous Ice Age, remaining constant until the beginning of the current interglacial period in which we live. This period began approximately 10,000 to 12,000 years ago.

During interglacial periods, steppe-tundra animals were challenged by both longer winters and their rapidly increasing range. These kinds of stresses encourage minor mutations in the gene pool of any species, resulting in subspecies that may eventually be reabsorbed into the DNA of the species as a whole.

A good example of this genetic phenomenon is the peregrine falcon. This raptor (bird of prey) has adapted to almost every environment on Earth, resulting in 27 subspecies that freely interbreed to produce hybrids. Even though each subspecies has different characteristics suited to its particular environment, all of the possible characteristics are contained in the DNA of each population of peregrines. Thus, when through their peregrinations (synonymous with "wanderings") these falcons find themselves in a new environment, they can rapidly evolve into subspecies that can efficiently adapt.

In the same way, a type of human that first arose in a previous interglacial period had a distinct advantage when confronted by the larger, harsher winters of the early part of the last Ice Age. This hominid species never developed the massive muscles evident in other hominids and apes. Because this new human's smaller muscle mass required less energy (at rest and under stress), more of the glucose obtained from carbohydrate foods was available for fat storage. The resulting fat storage was a valuable source of energy to this new human (in winter conditions and lean times). His more muscular relatives did not have access to such fat stores. The newly evolved hominid of the temperate steppe-tundra became increasingly common as the interglacial environment persisted into the early part of the last Ice Age.

During the last 70,000 years of intense glaciation this newly evolved hominid—i.e., modern man, *Homo sapiens sapiens* (Cro-Magnon)—came to dominate the gene pool. He thrived as the steppe-tundra moved closer to the equator. He also survived an event that led to the extinction of the world's largest game animals. Beginning approximately 40,000 years ago, this event is known as the Pleistocene Extinctions.

Virtually all of the large animals of the steppe-tundra became extinct before the steppe-tundra itself disappeared with the beginning of the current interglacial period. A few species such as wolves, bison, aurochs, and deer survived in small dry savanna or forest environments, but all of the larger species vanished. The refinements in technology that enabled *Homo sapiens sapiens* to exploit the megafauna species with which he evolved also enabled him to follow these animals to their extinction in the high Arctic. This polar route led him into the Western Hemisphere for the first time. Among the dry savanna and forest animal species that survived the Pleistocene Extinctions, only those that were domesticated during the beginning of the current interglacial warming period lived into the twentieth century at anywhere near their previous population levels.

Mesolithic Man

The hunters who made the difficult passage into the current interglacial period are known as Mesolithic (Middle Stone Age) or late Paleolithic humans. Their Ice Age origins left them with cravings for the meat of the fatty steppe-tundra grass eaters. Our intense cravings for sweets and our ability to rapidly convert carbohydrates to fat are legacies of our adaptation to the steppe-tundra climate.

The highly efficient hunting techniques of our steppe-tundra ancestors allowed them to survive in the environments that replaced the steppe-tundra. These seemingly simple hunting technologies allowed hunter-gatherers to live in places that, until the twentieth century, were uninhabitable to civilized, more technologically advanced people.

BIBLIOGRAPHY

Only through hunting and gathering knowledge will your path lead you to the meaning of life.

INTERNET RESOURCES

www.neanderthin.com—offers information, recipes, an E-mail link to the authors, and other useful resources for the *NeanderThin* convert. This web site will evolve according to the needs of those who visit the site.

www.panix.com/~paleodiet—provides links to Paleolithic nutrition research and related topics.

ARTICLES

Abrams, Jr., H. Leon, "Vegetarianism: An Anthropological/Nutritional Evaluation." *Journal of Applied Nutrition*, vol. 32, #2 (1980), 53–87.

Aiello, Leslie C. and Peter Wheeler, "The Expensive Tissue Hypothesis: The Brain and the Digestive System in Human and Primate Evolution." *Current Anthropology*, vol. 36, #2 (April 1995), 199–221. Analyzes human gut morphology and how eating meat made us smart.

Ames, B. N., "Ranking Possible Carcinogenic Hazards." *Science* 236 (April 17, 1987), 271–80.

————, "Paleolithic Diet, Evolution and Carcinogens." *Science* 238 (December 18, 1987), 1633–34.

————, "Carcinogenic Risk Estimation." *Science* 240 (May 20, 1988), 1043–47. Series of articles by one of the leading authorities on the causes of cancer. Ames shows how common foods may pose a greater threat of cancer than some of the chemicals often labeled carcinogenic.

Ascherio, A., and W. C. Willet, "Health Effects of Trans-fatty Acids." *American Journal of Clinical Nutrition*, vol. 66: 4 Suppl. (October 1997), 1006S–1010S.

Atkinson, Mark A., and Noel K. Maclaren, "What Causes Diabetes?" *Scientific American* (July 1990), 62–71.

Bishop, Jerry E., "More Fatty Foods Are Backed in Test of Diabetic Diets." *The Wall Street Journal* (May 11, 1994).

Boehmer, Harald von, and Pawel Kisielow, "How the Immune System Learns about Self." *Scientific American* (October 1991), 74–81.

Bower, B., "The 2-Million-Year-Old Meat and Marrow Diet Resurfaces." *Science News* (January 3, 1987), 7.

Bryant, Vaughn, "I Put Myself on a Caveman Diet—Permanently." *Prevention*, vol. 31, No. 9 (1979), 128–37.

———, "Eating Right Is an Ancient Rite." *Natural Science* (January 1995), 216–21.

———, "Prehistoric Diets." *University Lecture Series, Texas A&M University* (November 28, 1979).

———, "The Paleolithic Health Club." *1995 Yearbook of Science and the Future* (1994), published by Encyclopedia Britannica, Inc., Chicago, 114–33. Vaughn Bryant is the head of the Department of Anthropology at Texas A&M University and is also a professor of biochemistry.

Centofanti, M., "Diabetes Complications: More Than Sugar?" *Science News*, vol. 148 (December 23, December 30, 1995), 421.

Cerami, Anthony, Helen Vlassara, and Michael Brownlee, "Glucose and Aging." *Scientific American* (May 1987), 90–96.

Cohen, Leonard A., "Diet and Cancer." *Scientific American* (November 1987), 42–48.

Dahlqvist, Arne, "Lactose Intolerance," *Nutrition Abstracts and Reviews* (August 1984), 649–58.

De Bakey, Michael, *Journal of the American Medical Association*, vol. 189 (1964), 655–59. Shows that there is no definitive connection between serum cholesterol levels and atherosclerotic disease.

Diamond, Jared, "The Worst Mistake in the History of the Human Race." *Discover* (May 1987), 64–66. Explains how the invention of agriculture caused war, disease, oppression, and the income tax.

————, "The Great Leap Forward." *Discover* (May 1989), 50–60. Describes the Neolithic Revolution.

Dolnick, Edward, "Beyond the French Paradox." *Health* (October 1992), 40. Explains why the French have a high-fat diet and very little heart disease.

Dunbar, Robin, "Foraging for Nature's Balanced Diet; Finding the Link Between Diet and Longevity Among Human and Animal Groups." *Focus* (August 31, 1991) 25.

Eaton, S. B., and Melvin Konner, "Paleolithic Nutrition: A Consideration of Its Nature and Current Implications." *The New England Journal of Medicine*, vol. 312, no. 5 (January 31, 1985), 283–89. An absolute *must-read*!!!

Evans, G. H. et al., "Association of Magnesium Deficiency with the Blood Lowering Effects of Calcium." *Journal of Hypertension*, vol. 8 (1990), 327–37.

Frisch, Rose E., "Fatness and Fertility." *Scientific American* (March 1988), 88–95.

Garg, Abhimanyu, M.B.B.S., M.D., et al., "Effects of Varying Carbohydrate Content of Diet in Patients with Non-Insulin-Dependent Diabetes Mellitus." *Journal of the American Medical Association*, vol. 271, no. 18 (May 11, 1994), 1421–28. Shows how a low-fat diet caused a rapid increase in LDL-cholesterol levels in insulin-resistant–i.e., overweight–patients.

Henry, Linda, "Wild Side: Bodybuilders Advance to Primitive Protein for Lean Muscularity." *Muscle & Fitness* (March 1994), 85.

Hopkins, Susan, "Eating the Caveman's High-Fiber Diet Can Be Healthy." *The Battalion*, vol. 74 no. 179 (Thursday, July 23, 1981), 1.

Johnson, Mary Ann, "The Georgia Centenarian Study: Nutritional Patterns of Centenarians." *The International Journal of Aging & Human Development*, vol. 34 (1) (1992), 57–76. Explains that hundred-year-olds typically eat high-fat diets.

Krajick, Kevin, "Waiter, There's a Fly in My Soup, and I Ordered the Cricket Salad." *Newsweek* (September 20, 1993), 59E.

Larkin, Marilynn, "Cave Cuisine." *Health* (November 1985), 37–38.

Leonard, William R., and Marcia L. Robertson, "Evolutionary Perspectives on Human Nutrition: The Influence of Brain and Body Size on Diet and Metabolism." *American Journal of Human Biology*, vol. 6 (1994), 77–88. Similar to Aiello's "Expensive Tissue Hypothesis . . . "

Lowenstein, Jerold M., "Who Ate What When." *Oceans* (June 1988), 72.

Lutz, W. J., "The Colonization of Europe and Our Western Diseases," *Medical Hypotheses*, vol. 45 (1995), 115–120.

BIBLIOGRAPHY

McKie, Robin, "Meaty Evidence: Steak Made Humans Smart." (quotes *Current Anthropology* journal) *London Observer Service* (January 14, 1995).

Mead, Nathaniel, "Don't Drink Your Milk!" *Natural Health* (July/August 1994), 70–73, 112.

Milton, Katharine, "Diet and Primate Evolution." *Scientific American* (August 1993), 86–93.

Molleson, Theya, "The Eloquent Bones of Abu Hureyra." *Scientific American* (August. 1994), 70–75.

O'Dea, Kerin, Ph.D., et al., "Impaired Glucose Tolerance, Hyperinsulinemia and Hypertriglyceridemia in Australian Aborigines from the Desert." *Diabetes Care*, vol. 11, no. 1 (January 1988), 23–29. Compares effects of urban life and hunter-gathering on Australian Aborigines.

Raloff, J., "High-Fat Diets Help Athletes Perform." *Science News*, vol. 149, no. 18 (May 4, 1996), 287.

———, "Obesity, Diet Linked to Deadly Cancers." *Science News*, vol. 147, no. 3 (January 21, 1995), 39.

Reiser, Raymond, "The Three Weak Links in the Diet-Heart Disease Connection." *Nutrition Today*, vol. 14 (1979), 22–28.

Rennie, John, "The Body Against Itself." *Scientific American* (December 1990), 107–15.

Richardson, Sarah, "Medicine Watch: A One-Two to the Brain." *Discover* (November 1994), 36–37.

Roach, Mary, "Advice from the World's Biggest Weight Experts: Their Gain Can Be Your Loss." *Health* (March/April 1993), 62–72. Describes the traditional, low-fat diet of Japanese sumo wrestlers.

Rosenberg, Steven A., "Adoptive Immunotherapy for Cancer." *Scientific American* (May 1990), 62–69.

Scientific American, Special Issue: "Life, Death and the Immune System." (September 1993), entire issue.

Scrimshaw, Nevin S., "Iron Deficiency." *Scientific American* (October 1991), 46–52. Explains how vegetarian diets lead to anemia, lethargy, and reduced IQ in children.

Serra-Majem, Lluis, et al., "How Could Changes in Diet Explain Changes in Coronary Heart Disease Mortality in Spain? The Spanish Paradox." *American Journal of Clinical Nutrition* (1995), 13515–13595.

Shaper, A. G., et al., "Cardiovascular Studies in the Samburu Tribe of Northern Kenya." *American Heart Journal*, vol. 63, no. 4 (April 1962), 437–42.

Shepard, Paul, "A Post-Historic Primitivism." For "The Wilderness Condition: Realia Conference on Environment and Civilization." Estes Park, Colo. (August 17–23, 1989). Hunter-gatherer philosophy for the modern man.

Sojka, J. E., and C. M. Weaver, "Magnesium Supplementation and Osteoporosis." *Nutrition Review*, vol. 53 (1995), 71–74.

Speth, John D., "Early Hominid Hunting and Scavenging: The Role of Meat as an Energy Source." *Journal of Human Evolution*, vol. 18 (1989), 329–43. Attempts to calculate the amount of meat and fat required for hominid survival.

Stahl, Ann Brower, "Hominid Dietary Selection Before Fire." *Current Anthropology*, vol. 25, no. 2 (April 1984), 151–68. Explains the constraints on human diet without fire.

Stefansson, Vilhjalmur, "Adventures in Diet, Part 1." *Harper's Monthly Magazine* (December 1935), 668–75.

———, "Adventures in Diet, Part II." *Harper's Monthly Magazine* (January 1936), 46–54.

———, "Adventures in Diet, Part III." *Harper's Monthly Magazine* (February 1936), 178–89.

Stipp, David, "The Way We Were: Our Prehistoric Past Casts Ills in New Light, Some Scientists Say." *The Wall Street Journal* (Wednesday, May 24, 1995), 1 and A6, col. 1.

Stuart, Anthony J., "Mammalian Extinctions in the Late Pleistocene of Northern Eurasia and North America." *Biology Review*, vol. 66, no. 4 (1991), 453–563.

Torrey, John C., and Elizabeth Montu, "The Influence of an Exclusive Meat Diet on the Flora of the Human Colon." *Journal of Infectious Diseases*, vol. 49 (1931), 141–76.

United Press International, "Anthropologist: Eat Like a Caveman and Live to 100." *The San Diego Union* (Saturday, October 14, 1989), C6.

Urgert, Rob, et al., "Separate Effects of the Coffee Diterpenes Cafestol and Kahweol on Serum Lipids and Liver Aminotransferases." *American Journal of Clinical Nutrition*, vol. 65 (1997), 519–24.

Wallis, Michael, "Anthropologist Vaughn Bryant Lost 30 Pounds (But Not His Health) Eating What the Cave Dwellers Ate." *People* (February 19, 1979), 103–4.

Washington, Harriet, "The Back to the Future Diet; Healthy Diet Habits of Traditional Cultures." *Harvard Health Letter* (June 1994), 6.

Wurtman, Richard J., and Judith J. Wurtman, "Carbohydrates and Depression." *Scientific American* (January 1989), 68–75. Explains the role of complex carbohydrates in mood swings.

Zane, Frank, "Bodybuilding Advisory: Train with Zane: Eating for Muscular Definition." *Muscle & Fitness* (December 1994), 226.

Zvelebil, Marek, "Postglacial Foraging in the Forests of Europe." *Scientific American* (May 1986), 104–15. Documents the Neolithic Revolution in Europe.

STEFANSSON (all-meat diet) STUDIES

Lieb, Clarence W., M.D., "The Effects on Human Beings of a Twelve Months' Exclusive Meat Diet." *Journal of the American Medical Association* (July 6, 1929), 20–22. Stefansson's famous year-long experiment with an all-meat diet at Bellevue Hospital in New York.

McClellan, Walter S., Henry J. Spencer, Emil A. Falk, and Eugene Du Bois, "Clinical Calorimetry: XLIII. A Comparison of the Thresholds of Ketosis in Diabetes, Epilepsy, and Obesity." *Journal of Biological Chemistry*, vol. 80 (1928), 639–52.

———, and Eugene F. Du Bois, "Clinical Calorimetry: XLV. Prolonged Meat Diets With a Study of Kidney Function and Ketosis." *Journal of Biological Chemistry*, vol. 87 (1930), 651–68.

———, Virgil R. Rupp, and Vincent Toscani, "Clinical Calorimetry: XLVI. Prolonged Meat Diets With a Study of Nitrogen, Calcium, and Phosphorous." *Journal of Biological Chemistry*, vol. 87 (1930), 669–80.

———, Henry J. Spencer, and Emil A. Falk, "Clinical Calorimetry: XLVII. Prolonged Meat Diets with a Study of the Respiratory Metabolism." *Journal of Biological Chemistry*, vol. 93 (1931), 419–34.

———, and Vincent Toscani, "Clinical Calorimetry: XLIV. Changes in the Rate of Excretion of Acetone Bodies During the Twenty-Four Hours." *Journal of Biological Chemistry*, vol. 80 (1928), 653–58.

Tolstoi, Edward, "The Effect of an Exclusive Meat Diet Lasting One Year on the Carbohydrate Tolerance of Two Normal Men." *Journal of Biological Chemistry*, vol. 83 (1929), 747–52.

———, "The Effect of an Exclusive Meat Diet on the Chemical Constituents of the Blood." *Journal of Biological Chemistry*, vol. 83 (1929), 753–58.

Torrey, John C. and Elizabeth Montu, "The Influence of an Exclusive Meat Diet on the Flora of the Human Colon." *Journal of Infectious Diseases*, vol. 49 (1931), 141–76.

BIBLIOGRAPHY

BOOKS

Ardrey, Robert, *African Genesis.* New York: Antheneum, 1961.

———, *The Hunting Hypothesis.* New York: Atheneum, 1976.

Atkins, Robert C., *Dr. Atkins' New Diet Revolution.* New York: M. Evans, 1992.

———, *Dr. Atkins' Super-Energy Diet.* New York: Bantam Books, 1977.

Bernstein, Richard K., M.D., *Dr. Bernstein's Diabetes Solution.* New York: Little, Brown, 1997.

Bruce, Scott, and Bill Crawford, *Cerealizing America: The Unsweetened Story of American Breakfast Cereal.* Boston & London: Faber and Faber, 1995. Details the history of breakfast cereal in America with a brilliant section on the history of Dr. John Harvey Kellogg as told somewhat fictitiously in the feature film *The Road to Wellville.*

Bryant, Vaughn, "The Paleolithic Health Club." *1995 Yearbook of Science and the Future.* Chicago: Encyclopedia Britannica (1994), 114–33.

Budiansky, Stephen, *The Covenant of the Wild: Why Animals Chose Domestication.* New York: William Morrow, 1992. Explains the role of neoteny (domestication) in the Neolithic Revolution and how it was as much a biological as a technological evolution.

Campbell, Ada Marie, Marjorie Porter Penfield, and Ruth M. Griswold, *The Experimental Study of Food.* 2nd ed. Boston: Houghton Mifflin, 1979.

Chaitow, Leon, *Stone Age Diet.* London: Optima, 1987.

Chatwin, Bruce, *The Songlines.* New York: Viking, 1987. Talks about the religion of Australian Aborigines in particular and hunter-gathering in general.

Cohen, Mark Nathan, *The Food Crisis in Prehistory: Overpopulation and the Origins of Agriculture.* New Haven: Yale University Press, 1977. How environmental changes led man to seek new food sources.

———, *Health and the Rise of Civilization.* New Haven: Yale University Press, 1993. How man's new food sources produced new diseases.

——— and G. J. Armelagos, *Paleopathology at the Origins of Agriculture.* New York: Academic Press, 1984.

Corballis, Michael, L., *The Lopsided Ape: Evolution of the Generative Mind.* Oxford: Oxford University Press, 1991. Talks about how the difference in left and right brain size affected the evolution of human behavior.

Crawford, Michael and Sheilagh, *What We Eat Today: The Food Manipulators vs. the People.* New York: Stein & Day, 1972.

Desowitz, Robert S., *New Guinea Tapeworms and Jewish Grandmothers: Tales of Parasites and People.* New York, Avon Books, 1981.

BIBLIOGRAPHY

Diamond, Jared, *The Third Chimpanzee: The Evolution and Future of the Human Animal.* New York: Harper Perennial, 1992.

DiPasquale, Dr. Mauro, *The Anabolic Diet.* Optimum Training Systems, 1995. Low-carbohydrate diet used by bodybuilders and professional wrestlers.

Eades, Michael R., M.D. *Thin So Fast.* New York: Warner Books, 1989.

―――, and Mary Dan Eades, M.D., *Protein Power.* New York: Bantam Books, 1995. Highly recommended. Explains how low-carbohydrate diets work, focusing especially on insulin resistance. Excellent chapters on ancient diet and cholesterol metabolism.

Eaton, S. Boyd, Marjorie Shostak, and Melvin Konner, *The Paleolithic Prescription.* New York: Harper & Row, 1988. Arose from the landmark 1985 article in *The New England Journal of Medicine.* Constitutes a very conservative approach to Paleolithic Nutrition.

Farb, Peter, and George Armelagos, *Consuming Passions: The Anthropology of Eating.* Boston: Houghton Mifflin, 1980.

Fieldhouse, Paul, *Food & Nutrition: Customs & Culture.* London: Croom Helm, 1986.

Gare, Fran, and Helen Monica, *Dr. Atkins' Diet Cookbook.* New York: Bantam Books, 1974.

Gasset, Jose Ortega y, *Meditations on Hunting.* New York: Charles Scribner and Sons, 1972. Modern ruminations on hunter-gatherer philosophy.

Gleick, James, *Chaos: Making a New Science.* New York: Viking Penguin, 1987.

Harris, Marvin, and Eric B. Ross, *Food and Evolution.* Philadelphia: Temple University Press, 1987. Note especially Chapter 8 entitled "The Preference for Animal Protein and Fat: A Cross-Cultural Survey," written by H. Leon Abrams, Jr.

―――, *Cannibals and Kings: The Origins of Cultures.* New York: Random House, 1977. The story of how the needs of crop species forced man to become civilized.

―――, *Good to Eat: Riddles of Food & Culture.* New York: Simon & Schuster, 1985.

Hunter, Beatrice Trum, *The Great Nutrition Robbery.* New York: Charles Scribner and Sons, 1978.

Lee, Richard B., and Irven Devore, *Man the Hunter.* Chicago: Alpine Publishing, 1968.

Mandelbrot, Benoit B., *The Fractal Geometry of Nature*. New York: W. H. Freeman, 1977.

McGee, Harold, *On Food and Cooking: The Science and Lore of the Kitchen*. New York: Collier Books, 1984.

Oelschlager, Max, *The Idea of Wilderness*. New Haven and London: Yale University Press, 1991. Explains how our agricultural view of nature affects the environment.

Price, Weston, *Nutrition and Physical Degeneration*.

Sauer, Carl, O., *Seeds, Spades, Hearths & Herds: The Domestication of Animals and Foodstuffs*. 2nd ed., Cambridge: MIT Press, 1969.

Shepard, Paul, *The Tender Carnivore and the Sacred Game*. New York: Charles Scribner and Sons, 1973. A manifesto concerning how agriculture and neoteny conspire to oppress humans and destroy the environment.

Sieden, Lloyd Steven, *Buckminster Fuller's Universe: An Appreciation*. New York & London: Plenum Press, 1989, 367–68.

Simopoulos, Artemis P., M.D., and Jo Robinson, *The Omega Plan*. New York: HarperCollins, 1998.

Spencer, Colin, *The Heretic's Feast: A History of Vegetarianism*. Hanover & London: University Press of New England, 1995.

Stefansson, Vilhjalmur, *Cancer: Disease of Civilization*. New York: Hill and Wang, 1960. Documents the unsuccessful search for cancer and other autoimmune disorders among hunter-gatherers.

———, *Hunters of the Great North*. New York: Harcourt, Brace, 1922.

———, *The Fat of the Land* (originally, *Not By Bread Alone*, 1946). New York: Macmillan, 1956. The definitive book on pemmican.

Stillman, Irwin Maxwell, M.D., D-IM, with Samm Sinclair Baker, *The Doctor's Quick Weight Loss Diet*. Englewood Cliffs, NJ: Prentice Hall, Inc. 1967.

Taylor, Nadine, M.S., R.D., *Green Tea: The Natural Secret for a Healthier Life*. New York: Kensington Books, 1998.

Trinkaus, Erik, and Pat Shipman, *The Neanderthals: Changing the Image of Mankind*. New York: Knopf, 1993.

Voegtlin, Walter L., M.D., FAPC, *The Stone Age Diet*. New York: Vantage Press, 1975. Relies on studies of ecology and the human digestive system to support the idea that humans are primarily carnivorous.

Winterhalder, Bruce, and Eric Alden Smith, *Hunter-Gatherer Foraging Strategies: Ethnographic and Archeological Analyses*. Chicago: University of Chicago Press, 1981.

BIBLIOGRAPHY

Wright, Robert, *The Moral Animal: Why We Are the Way We Are: The New Science of Evolutionary Psychology.* New York: Pantheon Books, 1994. Discusses how our hunting and gathering instincts are the evolutionary basis of our morality.

INDEX

INDEX

low-fat, high-complex-
carbohydrate, high-fiber, 6
dietary fat, 55–57, 65–67, 71–72, 78–79
and cardiovascular disease, 164–66
and metabolism, 167
dietary laws, in antiquity, 3
diet drugs, 20
digestive enzymes, 103
digestive problems, 5
digestive system, of humans, 27–28
diseases
autoimmune, 9, 14, 168–69
"of civilization," 18
immune system, 16, 17–18
infectious, 18
dogs
diet of, 18, 46, 169
evolutionary link to wolves, 36–39
pet, diseases of, 46
similarities to humans, 28, 29, 36,
169
domestication, of wolves, 38
dressings, vinaigrette, 131
dyspepsia, 5

eating disorders, 20
eating out, 79
ecocide, agriculture and, 172, 177–78
eggs, 83
deviled, 121
egg drop soup, Roman, 120–21
and green onions, 115
omega-3 enriched, 66
puffy omelet, 116
tuna salad with, and onions and
avocado, 127–28
vegetable juice omelet, 113
emphysema, 18
endometriosis, 17
endorphins, 104
"energy accounting," 10
environmental preservation, and
NeanderThin diet, 177–78
epilepsy, 16, 18
Eskimo diet, 8–9
essential fatty acids (EFA), 78, 79
evolution
of dogs, 36–39
of humans, 24–32, 170, 180–85

of plants, to adapt to human
cultivation, 42, 176–77
exercise, 175
aerobic, 88–89, 101
five-week program, 87–102
mental activity as, 175
expensive tissue hypothesis of brain
size, 27
extinctions, 172–73
eye dominance, 31

falcons, peregrine, 184
farming culture, diets of, vs. hunting-
gathering diets, 21–22
fat. See body fat; dietary fat
fat to total body weight ratio, of
hunter-gatherers, 34
favism, 47
fertility, and Neolithic Revolution, 43
fiber, 7
fire, 39, 41
fish, 59
baked, 139–40
fish oil, 66, 79
flaxseed, 66, 79
food
cravings, 51–52, 104, 105
irradiated, 173
mass production of, 3–4
new types of, discovered in
Neolithic Era, 41
nutrient composition of, 6
packaged, 4, 174
permitted and forbidden, in
Neanderthin diet, 57–60
raw, 173–74
food cravings, 51–52, 104, 105
food diary, 157–63
food pyramid, USDA, 6, 64, 177
fractals, 11–12
frittata, spinach, mushroom, and
bacon, 111–12
fruits, 57, 59, 69–70
forbidden, digestibility of, 170
wild vs. cultivated, 63–64, 78
Fuller, R. Buckminster, 10

gene pools, mutations in, 184
glucose, 56, 164

INDEX

ABOUT THE AUTHORS

Ray Audette is a falconer in Dallas, Texas. When not hunting or gathering, Ray lectures, consults, and writes about Paleolithic nutrition. Ray received a Bachelor of Science degree from the University of Texas in 1975. He is actively involved in the Texas Hawking Association and Mensa and is a board member of the Dallas Philosophers' Forum.

Troy Gilchrist has been Ray's assistant since graduating with a Bachelor of Arts degree in philosophy from the University of North Texas in 1994. He is a certified massage therapist and a professional guitarist and songwriter.